Total Body Breakthroughs

The World's Leading Experts reveal proven

HEALTH, FITNESS & NUTRITION

SECRETS

TO HELP YOU ACHIEVE THE BODY YOU'VE ALWAYS WANTED BUT COULDN'T HAVE UNTIL

NOW!

Published by CelebrityPress™, Orlando, FL
A division of The Celebrity Branding Agency®

Celebrity Branding® is a registered trademark
Printed in the United States of America.

ISBN: 978-0-9829083-7-2
LCCN: 2010941457

This publication is designed to provide accurate and authoritative information with regard to the subject matter covered. It is sold with the understanding that the publisher is not engaged in rendering legal, accounting, or other professional advice. If legal advice or other expert assistance is required, the services of a competent professional should be sought. The opinions expressed by the authors in this book are not endorsed by CelebrityPress™ and are the sole responsibility of the author rendering the opinion.

Most CelebrityPress™ titles are available at special quantity discounts for bulk purchases for sales promotions, premiums, fundraising, and educational use. Special versions or book excerpts can also be created to fit specific needs.

For more information, please write:

CelebrityPress™,
520 N. Orlando Ave, #44,
Winter Park, FL 32789

or call 1.877.261.4930

Visit us online at www.**CelebrityPressPublishing**.com

Total Body Breakthroughs

The World's Leading Experts reveal proven

HEALTH, FITNESS & NUTRITION

SECRETS

TO HELP YOU ACHIEVE THE BODY YOU'VE ALWAYS WANTED BUT COULDN'T HAVE UNTIL

NOW!

TABLE OF CONTENTS:

FOREWORD
BY DAX MOY... 13

CHAPTER 1
THE SUCCESS MINDSET
BY ALWYN COSGROVE... 15

CHAPTER 2
KETTLEBELL TRAINING – BJ AND KORI'S STORY
BY B.J. BLIFFERT 27

CHAPTER 3
ACE LIVING TO OVERCOME ANY OBSTACLES
BY DAVID LEE.. 35

CHAPTER 4
KETTLEBELL FAT LOSS BLUEPRINT
BY JAMIE LLOYD.. 41

CHAPTER 5
**NOT YOUR TYPICAL 'FAT KID TO FITNESS
PHENOMENON' STORY**
BY BEN WARSTLER 51

CHAPTER 6
A FRESH NUTRITION PARADIGM
BY JON LE TOCQ.. 59

CHAPTER 7
**SECRETS TO STAYING ON TRACK DURING
WEIGHT LOSS**
BY KIM CHASE 67

CHAPTER 8
**MENTAL TOUGHNESS: THE KEY TO YOUR
FITNESS SUCCESS**
BY PAT RIGSBY 75

CHAPTER 9
WOMEN, MAKE YOUR BREAKTHROUGH
– SPECIFIC STRATEGIES FOR WOMEN TO MAKE A BREAKTHROUGH
BY RACHEL COSGROVE 83

CHAPTER 10
**PLAY FITNESS... THE TRUE ESSENCE OF MEGA-FAT
BURNING & 'KICK-ASS SHAPE' FOR LIFE**
BY BRIAN GRASSO 93

CHAPTER 11
'DEATH CAMP'
BY MARC KENT 103

CHAPTER 12
FROM FAT KID TO FIT PRO
BY STEVE KREBS.. 111

CHAPTER 13
**KETTLEBELL TRAINING FOR THE
FITNESS PROFESSIONAL**
BY PAMELA MACELREE 119

CHAPTER 14
THE DIFFERENCE BETWEEN SUCCESS AND FAILURE
BY JOHN O'CONNELL.. 125

CHAPTER 15
YOUR MIND/BODY EXPERIENCE
BY GREG JUSTICE, MA.. 133

CHAPTER 16
TIME MANAGEMENT AND A HEALTHY LIFESTYLE
BY NICK BERRY 141

CHAPTER 17
THE MIND: UNDERSTAND THE GREAT POWER WITHIN YOU – UNDERSTANDING PRECEDES CHANGE
BY JUSTIN YULE.. 149

CHAPTER 18
HOW TO MAKE FITNESS FUN! WELL, BETTER THAN FUN...TRULY REWARDING.
BY NIKI DAVIS... 161

CHAPTER 19
GETTING BETTER WITH BANDS!! – A RESISTANCE BAND TRAINING TRANSFORMATION
BY DAVE SCHMITZ.. 169

CHAPTER 20
FIVE STEP ACTION PLAN TO WIN THE FAT LOSS GAME
BY RYAN KETCHUM.. 177

CHAPTER 21
THE LAST MINUTE BEACH BODY
– A BLUE PRINT FOR BUSY PEOPLE LOOKING TO DROP BODY FAT, LOSE INCHES AND TONE UP IN ONLY 14 DAYS
BY JOE CARABASE 187

CHAPTER 22
BUILDING A BETTER MEAL PLAN
BY JAYSON HUNTER AND JIM LABADIE.. 201

CHAPTER 23
HOLISTIC WEIGHT LOSS STRATEGIES
BY STEVE JACK.. 213

CHAPTER 24
WHERE TO BEGIN WHEN YOU WANT TO LOSE 140LBS+
BY JULIA KNIGHT 225

CHAPTER 25
MISSION: METABOLISM
DISCOVER HOW TO FIX THE 7 DEADLY WORKOUT SINS TO ACHIEVE
METABOLIC BREAKTHROUGH
BY BJ GADDOUR... 233

CHAPTER 26
NUTRITION SUPPLEMENTS
BY JAYSON HUNTER... 253

CHAPTER 27
**ABS UNCRUNCHED – HOW TO GET A FLAT STOMACH
WITHOUT EVER DOING A SINGLE CRUNCH**
BY SCOTT COLBY 261

CHAPTER 28
THREE THINGS TO BUILD YOUR BODY NATURALLY
BY TYLER ENGLISH, NASM-PES, CPT, YFS 273

FOREWORD

BY DAX MOY

As a health and fitness professional with over a decade of education about what it really takes to get people into great shape fast and help them stay that way in the long-term, and a fairly decent reputation for delivering results to my own clients, I like to think I'm a good judge of what works and what doesn't when it comes to training, nutrition and motivation.

Every single week, I'm asked to endorse at least one product from a personal trainer or nutritionist who's trying to make a name for themselves in the fitness world and, unfortunately, every single week I'm forced to say no after reading their books or watching their videos.

It's not necessarily that they're bad, it's just that they're not good, or more correctly, not good enough.

Most fitness books tend to be written by people who have been in the fitness industry for only 5 minutes, and who still hang on to many of the fallacies about fat loss and getting into shape that the public does. Others tend to be same-old, same-old, 'me-too' versions of older, better books with nothing new or genuinely unique added to them.

Yet others still are just full of 'flaky' ideas and concepts that are based upon delivering short-term, quick-fix solutions that come at the expense of a person's long-term health and fitness, often leading to more of the very same problems that the books are supposed to be solving in the first place!

As you can appreciate, those aren't the kind of works that I'd be happy giving my stamp of approval to and feel good about. And hey, if you're not going to feel good about it, what's the point?

And so, I was asked to write the forward and endorse this book *Total Body Breakthrough* and initially expected to have to make my apologies in the usual manner. However, I was pleasantly surprised to find that not only was it put together by many of the rising stars in health, fitness and body transformation, but that it also had a slew of bona fide world-class experts chipping in as well!

Better still, it wasn't just a rehash of old material I'd heard over and over again, but rather it was all completely new ground-breaking material that most of the general public is unaware of.

The combined approach of tackling mindset, nutrition AND exercise in the way that it's covered in *Total Body Breakthrough* makes this a sure-fire hit that's bound to help anyone who uses it to get results faster and keep them longer than ever before... if they use it!

Everyone knows that you don't get amazing health and fitness results by reading a book, even one written by experts, you have to apply what you've read in EXACTLY the way you're told to, and without exception.

If you can do that, if you can read and you can follow instructions, I promise you, you'll experience results like never before. I can't promise they'll be easy (great results rarely come without great effort), but they'll come faster than you'd ever have expected... and they'll stay! Get ready for great results!

Dax Moy
The UK's Leading Personal Trainer
Author Of *The Magic Hundred Goal Achievement Program* and *The Look Great Naked Challenge*

Dax Moy
The UK's Leading Body Transformation Coach
http://www.londonpersonaltrainingstudio.com

Author Of *The Best-Selling MAGIC Hundred Goal Achievement Program*
http://www.themagichundred.com

Join my FREE Online Community TODAY at
http://www.daxmoy.ning.com

CHAPTER I

THE SUCCESS MINDSET

BY ALWYN COSGROVE

T wo shoe salesmen from competing companies were assigned to a new territory where neither company had ever been before. A little town in the middle of the jungle in Africa.

The first shoe salesman arrived after a long flight and started touring the town. He immediately called back to his office and demanded that he speak to his boss. "I can't believe what I'm seeing boss, this is an absolute waste of time, nobody here even wears shoes".

The second shoe salesman arrived after a similarly long flight, dropped his bags off and toured the town. It was within the hour that he too called back to the company and demanded to speak to his boss. "I can't believe what I'm seeing boss, this is an absolutely amazing opportunity, nobody here even wears shoes".

Hopefully you can see the point in my little story. When confronted with the same situation, one person sees the obstacles and one person sees the opportunity. The only difference is in how they interpret the situation. In other words, it's their mindset that makes the difference.

MY STORY

I started my sports training career as a competitive martial artist. I learned and honed my craft in a dingy high school gym hall in Scotland from a man called Derek Campbell. Always referred to as Mr. Campbell by the way....

My desire to continually improve was never ending. This quest took me to college to learn new, more effective methods of conditioning, and preparation for tournaments. It drove me to move overseas to seek out some of the World's best coaches, trainers and exercise science pioneers to enhance my fighting career.

Little did I know that the biggest fight of my life was just around the corner. And despite all the research I'd done, my success or failure was going to come down to how well I applied the lessons learned from my very first instructor.

THE FIGHT

In 2004, I had moved to Los Angeles, retired from competition and was married and running a gym.

However, something was not right. My ambition had gone, I was tired all the time, I was so inactive that I was gaining weight, I was depressed and my whole body hurt.

Eventually I went to the doctor for a battery of tests. Nothing came back. About a month or so later when going back to see the doctor, I noticed a lump in my thigh when I was in the shower. I assumed it was a muscle tear or an old injury that I'd aggravated.

We decided that we should do an ultrasound to see what it was. The ultrasound results came back inconclusive so we went to do a biopsy.

On July 27th 2004 I was given the results. Stage IV cancer. My body was riddled with the disease.

For the next six months, I was bombarded with chemotherapy and other interventions. I did 18 cycles of chemotherapy, each one lasting about 6-8 hours.

In Feb 2005 I was told that I was in full remission. I stopped chemo and tried to go on with my life.

But I was still tired. I never really got my energy back. And by the end of the year, I had severe back pain and spent most of my time lying on my back, with heat packs on my spine.

In Feb 2006 after my one year check-up PET/CT scan it turned out I had relapsed. And relapsed completely – once again I was in Stage IV (for those of you who don't understand this, with cancer there is no stage 5 – stage 5 is dead).

And so we entered the "second round" of the toughest fight of my life. This time we only did four rounds of chemotherapy. However, with much stronger drugs and each round lasted 144 hours (or 6 straight days).

At the end of these rounds I was given a stem cell/bone marrow transplant. June 13th 2006 I was in complete remission. This time for good.

LESSONS

So why am I telling you this in a book about exercise and transforming your body?

Because your success at undertaking this endeavor hinges almost entirely on your mindset. And I truly believe that my success in facing the biggest challenge of my life came down to my mindset. It had to – the doctors and nurses do their best and administer the same treatment to every patient that presents themselves with this disease. Yet some don't make it.

And it's the same with the exercise information in this book. The information is going to be the same for everyone who invests in this program. However, some people will have amazing results, and some people won't. It's all about how you take in and process that information – do you see the opportunities, or do you see the obstacles?

I believe the lessons I learned from my Taekwondo instructor back in the day saved my life and can be applied to anything.

1. MINDSET

It all starts with attitude. I don't know if you've ever bought a car and thought you were the only one in your area with that make and color. But then in the next few weeks -- you see the exact same color, make and model all over the place.

The truth is those cars were likely always there. Your mind just wasn't programmed to see them. Once you started to program your mind about this car -- you were aware how many were always around you.

Success is the same. Once you program your mind for success, you start to act differently, think differently and see opportunities that were always there, but your mind was blind to them before.

Read the following:

successfulchangeisnowhereinthisbook

I first saw this example of a mindset test on a TV show years ago, and was reminded of it recently, by New Zealand-born, UK-based, mind, body and energy coach Steve Jack, at a seminar at which we both presented.

You read one of two versions of the above.

1. Successful Change is Nowhere In This Book
   Or
2. Successful Change is Now Here In This Book

In other words, you were presented with the same information. Your mind (and your mindset) interpreted the information either positively or negatively based on it's programming. The cool part of all of this is that if you interpreted the wording in a negative form you can change the programming and start seeing success.

My childhood hero was Olympic Gold medalist and World Champion in five different weight classes – Sugar Ray Leonard. Leonard faced the best of the best and lost only 3 times in a career spanning 20 years (notably – his only loss by TKO came after a six-year lay off).

I can remember staying up in the middle of the night as a young kid to watch Leonard fight. I can even remember listening to a radio broadcast at about 4:00 am in Scotland, of the commentary on one of his fights. And then having to get up for school a few hours later!

I can also vividly recall an in-depth interview that he did, from his training camp, prior to one of his fights where the reporter asked:

"...if you were to take a beating...."

Ray cut him off -- shaking his head-- *"No. Next question."*

The reporter asked again: *"You won't talk about this?"*

Ray shook his head.

Reporter: *"Why not?"*

Leonard: *"Because it's not true"*

Reporter: *"You never will?"*

Leonard shook his head again.

Now, some people will think of this as pre-fight 'hype' or arrogance. I didn't see that. I saw a fighter so convinced of his readiness, of his will to win, and his ability to succeed that he could not comprehend defeat and was unwilling to even discuss the possibility.

Do you have that same mindset? When you start a project, are you *convinced* that you'll succeed? When you begin a fat-loss program, do you envision yourself lean and in great shape? Or does the self-doubt creep in? Success has to start from within.

"You have to know you can win. You have to think you can win. You have to feel you can win." – Sugar Ray Leonard

Here's a little 'quiz' that my TKD instructor taught me years ago. It's about fighting and apparently no top fighter ever gave a different answer. It ties in with the mindset of success.

"Picture two fighters engaged in combat. After a long tough battle, the one who has been slightly dominant catches the other in a chokehold and begins to tighten his hold. ...What would you do in that situation?"

Every champion fighter answered the same... "I'd keep squeezing until the other guy tapped out or went out!"

You see, a champion fighter just cannot picture that he (or she) is not winning the fight. It's inconceivable to them that they wouldn't succeed.

They feel that success is an inevitable conclusion. They don't lose. Ever. Not even for a second.

Most people instantly picture themselves as the one being choked. They immediately associate themselves with losing.

The champions couldn't even fathom that not winning was even an option.

This is the mindset that you need when you start training, start a new diet, want to burn fat and lose weight, start a business venture, or begin anything. Expect success to the point that anything but, is impossible for you to even imagine.

All those clichés are true: 'Where the mind goes, everything follows' and 'If you think you can or you think you can't – you're right'.

Step one: Expect success. When I was facing cancer I expected to win. No ifs, ands or buts. Regardless of percentages – I knew I was going to make it.

2. HABITS & BEHAVIORS

Noted author Michael Heppell once said, "Quick math problem -- Five frogs are sitting next to a pond on a hot day. One frog decides that the heat is getting too much and decides to jump into the cool water. How many frogs are left?"

Now if you answered four – you're wrong. You see, there are still five frogs because deciding to do something is only step one. Nothing changes until you actually take action.

Are your daily behaviors getting you closer to, or further from, your goals.

Write down everything you do each day for a week, and take a good honest look at some of your activities and habits. Are they congruent with a successful person? What does a successful person on an exercise program do when they get up in the morning? Where do they go? Who do they talk to? What do they think? How many books or educational DVD's have they studied? How much time did they spend listening to educational material while traveling, as opposed to listening to music or talk radio?

Make sure your mindset is not being sabotaged by less successful behaviors.

When facing cancer I had to get my mind right – but we also had to take tangible action towards getting well. My doctors and nurses helped me – but I still had to do things.

Take action towards your goals every day.

My instructor taught me – you're either getting better or getting worse. You're either getting closer to your goals or further away. There is no standing still – the body is way too complex for nothing to be happening. When you face your goal, you can only reach it by constant forward progress.

 In the hospital I drank my water, took my vitamins, ate my food, and got up to exercise every single day – even when I was tired and vomiting. I knew I had to take action.

Every little thing you do, regardless of how insignificant it is, gets you closer to your intended result or further away. Take positive action!

3. SHARPENING

This is about developing more skills or getting more education -- or just sharpening and 'plain getting better' at what you already know and do.

What do you need to know about how to do? What separates you from someone who is being more successful than you? I can guarantee it's either education or skills.

Do you know everything that's needed to get to the next level? If not, start identifying your weak areas and get to work on them.

Reading constantly is a great way to grow. Even if the book is heavy going and you don't understand some of it -- there is still information sinking in at some level. You are still growing because of it.

And don't be afraid to re-read this book or your notes, over and over again. Pull your old notes off the shelf and get to work reviewing them. Remember education is about "self help" not "shelf help".

I heard someone say something at a seminar last year that I had already heard (and on some level knew), that I immediately put into action. It was a good reminder for reviewing stuff you've already studied.

"You can't solve a problem with the same mind that created it."

Every great fighter, no matter what level they are at, has a coach and training partners to get them to the next level.

In my cancer experience – I asked questions and educated myself on things I could do to help fight the disease. I talked to survivors. I read Lance Armstrong's book. I kept trying to get better and better.

4. ENVIRONMENT

This is about masterminding, seminars you attend, colleagues you talk to, and even your social life.

When you surround yourself with people who are going someplace, you are 99% more likely to go with them.

Mark Victor Hansen (author of *Chicken Soup For The Soul*) has said: "Your income, the results you create, are dictated by the five people you spend the most time with."

If you keep goldfish, or other tropical fish – when the fish are sick, what's the first thing you do to get them better? You change the water.

You don't treat the fish. You treat the environment. You make it better.

In order to reach your goals, you need to make sure you have a supportive environment. Do you have a partner in this journey? Do you have a good trainer who is helping you? Does your gym allow you to get access to the tools you need on your journey?

Every champion has a support team – an environment – that lives and breathes success. Change your environment if you're not getting to your goal fast enough. My instructor changed my sparring partners or drills any time I was getting stale.

After my first cancer experience, I changed doctors – as my first doctor wasn't, in my opinion, positive enough. I emailed people about my experiences and whittled the email list down to only the people who I felt were positive influences.

5. CHUNK IT DOWN

I can remember having to face a scary opponent in a championship match once. This guy was on the covers of all the martial arts magazines and this was my first time competing in this weight class. He was bigger, stronger and more experienced than I was.

In short, I was terrified. My instructor, Mr. Campbell, recognized this and asked me –

"I know you're scared. On a scale of one to ten, how scared are you?"

I answered with no hesitation " TEN!"

He smiled and said – "Ok. How scared would you be if this match was only one round in length?"

I answered, "Not as scared. Maybe a seven out of ten."

He said "Well keep that in mind. You only have to fight the first round. But what if the first round was only one minute long? Would you still feel the same way?"

Me: "No. That would maybe be a five out of ten."

Mr. Campbell nodding: "Ok. What if it was just a single exchange in the middle of the ring? One time. Then it's over. How do you feel about that?"

Me: "Ha! No problem. Maybe one out of ten. I'm too fast for him if it's a single exchange!"

Mr C: "Ok – let's just attack once and then we'll take it from there."

At this point I'm buzzing with excitement, stepped into the ring and attacked my opponent. And just repeated that single activity over and over. No fear at all.

And I won the fight.

Fitness is similar. Losing 50 or 60 lbs can seem overwhelming. But if I broke it down into one 10 lb goal at a time it becomes a lot easier to achieve. So ten pounds in the first five weeks is our goal – which means we need to lose 2 lbs of fat per week.

This means we need to exercise for 3-4 hours this week, eat supportive meals 90% of the time (we don't need perfection), and make sure you are well hydrated.

Which means: today – go the gym and eat 5 good meals – one meal every few hours.

Which means: now – go get a glass of cold water and print out your program for today's workout.

Now you can do that, right?

Of course. Now just do it again….

In the hospital after my transplant, I knew the day I could be discharged depended on my white blood count. I marked off on a calendar every day that I was one step closer, and put a graph together of my WBC every single day – every time I looked at it, I was one step closer. And soon enough I was being allowed to go home!

SUMMARY

You are about to embark on a journey. You've been given the same map and same instructions as everyone else. But everything depends on your mindset and attitude.

I'll see you at the end of the journey!

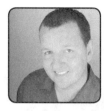

ABOUT ALWYN

Born in Scotland, and initially exposed to fitness training through an intense competitive sport martial arts background, Alwyn Cosgrove began reading and studying any training related material he could get his hands on. This led Alwyn to formal academic studies in Sports Performance at West Lothian College. He then progressed to receive an honors degree in Sports Science from Chester College, the University of Liverpool.

During his career as a fitness coach, Alwyn began with assisting in martial arts lessons in 1986, and teaching fitness classes in 1989. He has studied under all of the top fitness professionals and coaches in the world. Alwyn has also worked with a wide variety of clientele, from general population clientele to several top-level athletes, World Champions and professionals ⬚ in a multitude of sports.

A sought after 'expert' for several of the country's leading publications, including as a regular contributor to Men's Health magazine, Alwyn has co-authored three books in the "New Rules of Lifting" series. He currently spends his time training clients, training his staff at Results Fitness, speaking on the lecture circuit, and coaching fitness trainers worldwide in their businesses.

For the past decade, along with his wife Rachel, Alwyn runs Results Fitness in Santa Clarita, California ⬚ which has been named three times one of America's Top Gyms by Mens Health magazine; it is a gym which specializes in programs for real-world busy people, and prides itself on "changing the way fitness is done – period!"

You can reach Alwyn at www.alwyncosgrove.com

CHAPTER 2

KETTLEBELL TRAINING – BJ AND KORI'S STORY

BY B.J. BLIFFERT

I became interested in fitness in high school. I was always "stocky", but short, and wanted to get a little bigger and stronger. I started lifting weights after school and really enjoyed it, and because of my frame and build I saw increases in size and strength very quickly.

Funny thing. During college, although I was still training, I was considerably less active. I started to notice I was gaining quite a bit of weight and not all of it good. Although I was still lifting weights, I quickly went from stocky, to husky, to fat.

After College I knew if I wanted to get a job as a Fitness Pro I needed to "get in shape". Being strong, but fat, wasn't going to cut it.

In 2001, while paging through a magazine, I came across kettlebell training. The kettlebell was touted as the "secret" fitness tool of the Russian Military, used to create a strong lean body with everlasting cardio. I thought "what the heck", and ordered one.

After my first training session, while lying on the ground gasping for air, I knew this was the tool for the results I had been trying to achieve.

Almost overnight my bodyfat dropped, it seemed like I flipped the 'fat burning' switch. My body was transforming FAST. I didn't weigh myself often, but I was consistently over 200 pounds (I'm only 5'6"). Since discovering kettlebell training, I walk around at a comfortable and fit 165.

KORI'S STORY:

From the time I was 8 years old I was fat. Or as some people would say, I had a pretty face or a great personality. I was and still am, a "big portion girl". I LOVE FOOD!!! And not only that, I am an emotional eater. I use food to cope with just about any emotion. Happy, sad, mad or frustrated, food helps me celebrate or just get through it.

I remember my parents trying to help me eat better by the age of 10, nudging me toward sports and/or exercise. My mom was an overweight child, so she knew the troubles that lay ahead. But, I wasn't ready and kept my habit of eating junk food. It wasn't until I didn't make the cheerleading squad in eighth grade that I paid attention to my predicament, because I couldn't do most of the jumps and flips because of my weight. I started using starvation diets and doing my mom's aerobic tapes. My weight yo-yo'd up and down during the next few years.

In college I started using diet pills. The large amounts of caffeine in these pills curbed my appetite and I lost weight without even exercising. My weight continued to yo-yo throughout college. I just figured that was how it was going to be.

I never weighed myself at my heaviest. All I know is that in my last year of college I wore a size 16 and they were extremely tight.

After college I met BJ, he helped me understand I'd have to exercise and eat properly to maintain a healthy weight. He designed a program for me using kettlebells. The change was noticeable within two weeks. I went from 145 to129 pounds, from size 8 to size 4 jeans within two months. I knew then I wanted to become a fitness professional, and help women lose weight and be healthy and strong – without crazy starvation diets and diet pills that make you want to climb walls!!

We're going to show you how you can use the kettlebell to achieve the results you read about above.

1. LEARN PROPER TECHNIQUE

I realize it sounds like Kori and I jumped right in and instantly got fantastic results. It needs to be mentioned that we were both very active and had been practicing the exercises with dumbbells before our first kettlebell arrived. Even then, it took about two weeks to become comfortable with these new exercises.

The great thing about kettelbell training is that just learning and practicing the exercises, in the beginning, will serve as your workout. This is truly a "learn-by-doing" activity.

2. KEEP IT SIMPLE

In the beginning there is no need to get fancy, in fact, you'll start with only one exercise, the kettlebell swing. In total we work with three exercises, the swing, the snatch and the clean & jerk (or it's complicated cousin, the clean & press). We realize this doesn't sound like a lot, but these exercises are chosen for the large amount of muscle mass used to perform them. You'll burn maximum calories in minimum time. Simple. Effective. Efficient.

3. START SLOW

Just like starting any new exercise program, start slow. If you were to start a running program, you wouldn't start by running a marathon. Take your time and learn the movement correctly and safely. You'll notice very quickly this is unlike any other fitness program you have tried. Starting slow and taking your time and exercising within your limits, insures steady progress.

4. ONE KETTLEBELL, ONE CLOCK OR TIMER.

In the beginning this is all you need. Since this is a new skill that you will be "practicing" you'll need more rest in the beginning to ensure you don't develop any bad habits.

To start, take your clock (you'll need one with a second hand) and at the top of every minute, perform 5 Two-Arm Kettlebell Swings. You'll continue to do this until your technique is an 8 on a scale of 1-10. That may be 5 minutes or it maybe 10. Right now it doesn't matter, once your technique is an 8, you're done for the day.

Work your way up to 20 minutes, adding on 1-2 minutes per workout, given your technique is sound. Your goal is to work up to 20 repetitions on the top of each minute for twenty minutes. This will roughly translate to 30 seconds of work with 30 seconds of rest. 3 days a week seems to work best.

5. PRACTICE NEW SKILLS AS PART OF YOUR WARM UP.

After 4-6 weeks of kettlebell swings, and you are comfortable with the movement, you can start to add in other movements. BUT, since these are new, we are going to start the same way we did a few weeks earlier when we learned the swing.

So, after some stretches, mobility drills and some basic calisthenics, like push ups and squats, practice either the Kettlebell Snatch or Kettlebell Clean & Jerk/Press as the second part of your warm up, once you get comfortable with them. This will further warm up the hips, upper back and shoulders, preparing you for your swings and making it easier to transition into these drills as the main part of your workout, once you have worked up to the prescribed 20 minutes above. You can see step-by-step demos and videos of these drills at the end of this chapter and on our blog at: http://fullthrottlefitnessblog.com.

One thing you'll notice right away is you're changing from a movement that requires two hands on the kettlebell to movements that only require one hand on the kettlebell. A good transition move is a One Arm Swing, this will strengthen your grip and get you ready for the intermediate movements.

Moving On...

As you become more and more proficiant with the Kettlebell Snatch and the Kettlebell Clean & Jerk/Press you can start to make them the primary movement in your fat loss program. You will quickly realize one major difference between these two movements and the Kettlebell Swings is there are certain points in the movement where you can "rest". For the Snatch, it is overhead and for the Clean & Jerk/Press it's both in the "rack" position and again overhead. Learning to take short breaks in these key spots will allow you to prolong the time the kettlebell is in your hand, thus increasing the number of calories you'll burn throughout your workout.

Using intervals of 30 seconds on the right arm, 30 seconds on the left arm, resting 30 seconds to one minute and then repeating this process as long as your technique is an 8 out of 10, ensures maximum caloric expediture in minimal time. We work up times as long as 30 minutes in this format. Like before, this can't be stressed enough: build up the length of your workouts slowly. In the beginning, if you feel you aren't getting enough out of the workout due to your skill level with these new exercises, add in some sets of swings afterward. This will keep your heart rate up and burn more calories.

As you progress and your fitness level increases, you can start to decrease the rest period between your sets, or increase the length of your set. Decreasing your rest period from one minute to 45 seconds may not seem like much, but you'll soon feel the effects. Likewise, increasing your work time from 30 to 45 seconds or even to one minute will greatly increase the number of repetitions you perform during your workouts. It is not uncommon to eventually eliminate the rest period all together and simply keep changing hands back and forth at set time intervals or after a specific number of repetitions. The key is to play around with this and make it challenging and fun.

These are big "bang for the buck" exercises, using a large number of muscle groups. Remember, we are after results, oftentimes the simpler we can make our workouts the easier they will be to stick to. This will lead to more consistency and consistency leads to lasting results.

TWO ARM SWING

1. Place 2 hands on the Kettlebell. Give the Kettlebell a small back swing like hiking a football.
2. As the Kettlebell reverses direction and starts to swing forward, drive your heels into the ground allowing the Kettlebell to swing forward, remember your arms are just tethers, DO NOT LIFT WITH YOUR ARMS. Extend your hips and allow your power to lift the Kettlebell.
3. As the Kettlebell reaches the desired height (above), reverses directions and starts back toward the starting position, once the

upper arms come in contact with the torso, fold at the hips by pushing the hips back (below) and allow yourself to sink back into the athletic squat position. The Kettlebell does not reset on or touch the deck. Think of "hiking" a football.

4. Repeat the hip extension to start the next swing. The Kettlebell will swing back and forth similar to a pendulum. Repeat for the prescribed number of repetitions or time interval.

ONE ARM SWING

Perform just as you did the Two-Arm Swing, but take one hand off the bell and add a slight "scooping" motion with the hips as illustrated on the website. This gives the Kettlebell some elevation and keeps it closer to the body, making it easier to transition to the snatch later on.

KETTLEBELL SNATCH

1. Start the Kettlebell Snatch the same as you would the One Arm Swing, but use a little more force allowing the kettlebell to elevate overhead in one motion where you will receive it in the "lockout" position, seen below.
2. After a brief pause, allow the kettlebell to move around the hand in a "corkscrew" motion where it will start the down swing.
3. The Kettlebell will swing down between the legs, again just like the One Arm Swing. Repeat this process for the set time or number of repetitions.

CLEAN & JERK/PRESS

1. Start the Kettlebell Clean & Jerk/Press the same as you would the One Arm Swing, by swinging the kettlebell back between the legs. As the kettlebell swings forward slightly "scoop" hips under the kettlebell to give the kettlebell some elevation and keep it close to your body.
2. With your upper arm close to your side, bend your elbow and allow the bell to move around your hand and land in the "V" created by your upper and lower arm as shown above. This is the Rack position. Try to create contact between your elbow and hip.
3. Slightly dip from your knees, and using your legs drive the kettlebell up as seen in the illistrations on the website. The

upward motion should come mainly from the legs, not the arm and shoulder.

4. As the kettlebell is traveling up, dip under the kettlebell by pushing the hips to the rear to straighten and lock the elbow. This will take pratice. You can view detailed videos and demos on our blog at http://fullthrottlefitnessblog.com. If you are unable to, or feel uncomfortable with this, you can eliminate this step and simply press the kettlebell overhead.

5. Lower the kettelbell back to the Rack position as seen here.

6. Swing the kettlebell back between the legs to start the next repetition. Repeat this process for the prescribed number of repetitions or time interval.

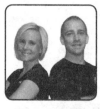

ABOUT BJ & KORI

The Full Throttle Kettlebell Program is the only one of it's kind in the Dallas Area, emphasizing authentic Russian techniques as they are taught in the Kettlebell's homeland using programs similar to those used to train the Russian Military. In May of 2011, BJ & Kori join the ranks of only a handful of American coaches to travel to St Petersburg, Russia to train with, and be trained by, Russian coaches and multiple-time World Champion Kettlebell athletes.

In addition, their Semi-Private and Youth Fitness training programs help clients of all ages make fitness a part of a healthy lifestyle.

BJ has a degree in Fitness Management and holds multiple certifications ranging from Strength and Conditioning to Kettlebell Training, Corrective Exercise and Nutrition.

Kori has a degree in Biology and also maintains certification in Personal Training, Kettlebell Training, Corrective Exercise and Nutrition.

To learn more about BJ & Kori and Full Throttle Athletics services, go to: http://fullthrottleathletics.com.

You can get a copy of their Free Special Report "7 Strategies to Finally get Lean and Mean" and get free 'cutting-edge' fitness and nutrition tips and 'how to' exercise videos at: http://fullthrottlefitnessbolg.com

CHAPTER 3

ACE LIVING TO OVERCOME ANY OBSTACLES

BY DAVID LEE

I t's hard to believe that it has been a little over ten years since my horrifying car accident. At the time I was a 'know-it-all' teenager and it nearly cost me my life. I hit a telephone pole going over ninety-five miles an hour and my life has never been the same since.

The three years following my accident were a living hell. I was told by my doctors that I would probably never be able to walk again, at least not without pain. I had broken my tibia and fibula in both legs, my left leg was so badly injured that they considered amputating it. I also shattered my femur and knocked out the majority of my upper jaw, which caused countless hairline fractures throughout my face.

During those years I had numerous surgeries. I had a plate, two rods and twenty-four screws inserted and removed from my legs. The most painful surgery was when they removed bone from my hip to do bone grafting. Once all this was in place, I had ACL and MCL surgeries in both knees.

I thought these were supposed to be greatest years of my life, but instead it was a living nightmare. The accident took place the summer between my freshman and sophomore years in college. Instead of participating in golf outings with high schools friends or tag football with college room-mates, I was a prisoner to my own body. I was chained to a hospital bed for weeks, shackled to a wheel chair for months, and 'cruised on crutches' for the remainder of my college career. To make matters worse, the doctors told me that physical activity was a thing of the past for me. I fell into a deep depression and gained over sixty pounds.

I was appreciative of the fact that I was still alive and walking, but I couldn't help but be angry at myself for what I had put myself through. Feeling numb to everything, I coasted through the years following my recovery. It was a difficult time in my life and I turned to alcohol to ease the pain. I was staying out till all hours of the night getting 'wasted' with friends; it was the one thing that didn't get handicapped during my ac-cident. It wasn't until six years later that I had an epiphany.

In late 2006, I met my beautiful wife. She helped me realize that I could not live the rest of my life in self-pity, for that wasn't living. I was at a crossroads, I could continue to live my life in self-loathing, or toughen up and make a change.

I choose the latter, I toughened up and made a change. I started off slowly by performing body weight exercises and working through the pain. I immediately felt the difference and in no time at all my friends and fam-ily noticed a change in my body, mind and attitude.

Everywhere I went people said things like, "Is that **YOU**?", "**YOU** look so good, David", "What have you been doing?" ...And most of all, "Can I do it with you?" And I said, "YES, of course you can!"

This is when I had my epiphany. I realized that I lived through my ac-cident to help others overcome their own obstacles and self-doubt, and to aid them in reaching their fitness goals. I took a risk and founded my own company, Real World Strength Coach LLC.

At first I took on only a few clients. I was still working forty-plus hours a week and scheduling was a bit of a hassle. I noticed that no matter how run-down I was, I always had energy for my clients. I couldn't help but feel like I was neglecting them in some capacity, so I took a giant leap of faith and quit my full time job – so that I might focus solely on my new business venture. It was scary, but I had never felt so invigorated; I knew it was my calling.

I've been doing what I love since 2007. I am proud of the change I've made within myself and my community. To ensure that I continue to make positive changes and stay on the right path, I follow the ACE way of life. ACE stands for Associate, Clean, and Elevate. To you these might be three meaningless words, but I will show you how living by these words will change your life for the better.

I founded ACE living when I quit my full time job. This way of life will undoubtedly allow you to fully 'maximize' from your life experiences. We, as a society, often go through the motions and don't take time to enjoy anything that is going on around us. By following these three easy steps, you will lead an overall more fulfilling, healthy and enriched life.

In order to start living the ACE way of life, you must first figure out who you are and who you want to be. You've heard it time and time again … you are a product of your environment. In order to be a positive product, you must first find an environment that you will thrive in. Three years ago, I looked at myself in the mirror and the person I saw was not who I wanted to be. I saw a miserable, depressed individual who was faking happiness through binge drinking and partying too much. I wanted to be an entrepreneur with a thriving business who is a positive, not negative, contributor to society.

I was lacking meaning in life. I had no purpose, no goals, no ambition – and I wanted more for myself and my future family. I knew that everything I had been through served a purpose... I just didn't know what at the time. It took me six years to realize that my accident, pain and suffering served as a foundation to help others who've experienced similar hardship.

Associating yourself with the right group of people is difficult, because most people want to see you fail. I know it sounds harsh and I am a totally 'glass-half-full' kind of guy, but that's just the way life is. The only way to ensure success is by putting the right systems in place and removing negative temptations that often lead to bad choices. Think about your worth and who you are and find people who have similar goals and the same desire to succeed. Distance yourself from those who bring you down and do not care about your growth; don't allow yourself to play into their negativity. Stay focused on the positive and good things will come your way.

Associating yourself with like-minded individuals is the first step in leading a more fulfilling life. The next step is easier said than done. Leading a cleaner lifestyle is challenging, especially in the society we live in. I will give you one tip though... if you are surrounded by others on the same path of life, it lowers temptation and increases the likelihood of your success. Many of my clients, whom I now consider family, are on the same wavelength as I. We began living and eating 'clean' for different reasons, but with one common goal ...to be healthier individuals.

The easiest way to succeed in leading a cleaner way of life is to follow two simple criteria when purchasing food. Next time you are at the market refrain from purchasing anything with [a] more than five ingredients, or [b] anything with a word that you cannot pronounce or don't know the meaning of.

Our bodies aren't meant to process many of the chemicals and bi-products that are in most store stocked items. It's about sticking to the natural stuff like fresh organic fruits and vegetables, cage-free eggs, grass-fed meats, raw milks and cheeses.

Leading a cleaner life will increase your energy levels and invigorate your life. But nothing will revitalize you like the last principal of ACE living. It's all about elevation. As we grow older I find that we settle for less more often. In other words we, as individuals, become content easier. This is why this principal is so important... if applied correctly you will find yourself doing things you never dreamed possible.

This step is easy, just remember to set realistic goals and continue to elevate them when they are reached. You can elevate just about anything ... elevate your work ethic, elevate your passion, elevate your drive, elevate your goals. These will all in turn elevate your life!

I remember when I was one of those people who complained about the workweek, "Ohhhh, its Monday again... kill myself" or "Gosh, I can't wait till Friday!" I was like a broken record; I would enjoy my weekends and then complain when Monday rolled around. I found myself complaining two hundred and sixty days out of the year; of course I was miserable! I was spending almost seventy-five percent of the year whining. This motivated me to do something I loved; it is one of the reasons I started my company.

Take a leap of faith and do something that brings you joy. Don't be someone who just waits for great things to happen; you must achieve what you've set out to accomplish. Don't be someone who settles for less; always keep your eye on the prize and don't give up till it's yours.

The elevation principle can easily be applied when it comes to fitness. How many people do you know that set a fitness goal as their New Year resolution? Countless, I bet. We live in a society of instant gratification. We want the results without putting in any of the work. I make sure that those I train are constantly elevating their training. It is important not to forget to continue challenging yourself in all aspects of life. Pushing yourself to the limit whenever possible will guarantee success in any goals you've set for yourself.

ACE has provided me with more time and energy to enjoy my growing family. These simple principles continue to stimulate me to achieve goals I set out for myself. They have made life much more enjoyable. ACE will undoubtedly continue to challenge me to be the best version of me possible: A better father for my newborn son, Justus Rafael; A better husband to my wife, Ana Lee; A better trainer for my clients; An overall better me – because it's all about elevating my standards and becoming the difference I wish to see in the world.

ACE living will change your life, and the life of those you love, for the better. It's simple, start by associating yourself with like-minded people. Continue by eating cleaner to increase your energy levels and life expectancy. Elevate everything you do. Give one hundred percent and don't settle for anything but what you've set out to achieve. ACE is a simple but effective way to better your life and I dare you to challenge yourself and enjoy life to the fullest. I look forward to associating with you one day.

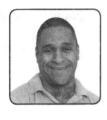

ABOUT DAVID

David Lee, owner of Real World Strength Coach LLC, CPT, YFS has over 5,000 hours helping local Philadelphians transform their lives through his ACE living principles (Associate, Clean, and Elevate) and No Excuses Training.

David got his start in the business due to a horrific car accident and his deep desire to get his body back in shape. Once he found his new life principles of ACE living, he was able to overcome the obstacles he faced after his accident. He realized that through these principles he could help others overcome their daily struggles, and get the body they always dreamed of.

Dave studied under Zach Even-Esh and started to perfect his training style. He made it his passion to learn all he could about bodyweight, kettlebell and metabolic training. He took his new-found knowledge and started up a small time fitness boot camp out of his home garage; there the Real World Strength Coach was born.

He continued to study, learn and transform his own body along with the lives of his clients. Within the next six months he left his full time job and opened his own warehouse training facility. Real World Strength Coach quickly became the place to go if you wanted a "real workout!"

Since then, David has helped numerous local Philadelphians, whom he now calls family, transform their lives and bodies. He has helped them lower cholesterol, drop diabetes numbers, reduce body fat, and improve overall body composition and self-image. Not only have his members witnessed physical changes, but they've had a life-changing experience that has allowed them to lead healthier lives.

Dave also serves as the strength and conditioning coach for two medal-winning Dragon Boat teams in the Philadelphia area. 'Hope A Float' is composed entirely of breast cancer survivors, together they inspire others. He has also worked first hand with the city's youth in hopes of stopping the escalating obesity problem. Dave was featured on Good Morning America Health, and is often recognized as Philadelphia's top fitness and weight loss expert.

Dave hopes to expand his facility so that he can help more individuals. He also plans on taking his ACE message to the world via his new website and blog.

David is married to Ana Lee, and has a three-month-old son with whom he is blessed to spend every day with. There is no doubt that with the passion and drive he encompasses, he will be able to influence countless lives for the better.

CHAPTER 4

KETTLEBELL FAT LOSS BLUEPRINT

BY JAMIE LLOYD

A typical day for me includes chugging green drinks and swinging kettlebells between personal training appointments, but it wasn't always like this. Back in my 20s, life was a bit different. Growing up in Wales, I burned the candle at both ends, playing rugby and looking forward to socialising with the team after a match. My idea of nutrition was whatever I could find in my fridge.

But when I gave up rugby, my passion for fitness stayed. I took up long-distance running, triathlon and duathlon but it wasn't long before a back injury I'd picked up playing rugby told me it was time to stop. Just 18 months ago, I had chronic sciatica. Treatment included cortisone injections, muscle relaxants and lots of painkillers. I was at an all-time low: I could barely walk, gained 14 lbs, and developed a 'beer belly'.

Something had to give.

The fact is, I realised training hard wasn't enough to give me the lean body I wanted. I was constantly tired, felt lethargic and was over my ideal bodyweight. The final straw came when I took a good look at myself and realised I was one of the least healthy personal trainers out there.

It wasn't good enough.

After back surgery, I decided to embark on a major personal health-kick. I wanted to reclaim my health, take control and feel like I was 20 years old again.

What did I do? I took an intensive course in yoga (what would my rugby mates have thought of that?), did light kettlebell training and followed an alkalising diet. This consisted of eating clean, eliminating man-made foods and introducing organic whole foods. I also drank filtered water at least 80% of the time. The results were great, and now I'm passionate about educating other people.

I see the same problems with many of my personal training clients. They usually arrive in a poor state of health. Many are overweight and some are at crisis point. I put together my "Kettlebell Fat Loss Blueprint" to help guide them all the way. Now you can get the same results, because I'm going to give you the "Kettlebell Fat Loss Blueprint." (…along with some extras!)

Follow my tips just 80% of the time and you'll be healthier, fitter and happier. I know, because I've been following it myself and I have more energy, my eczema has cleared up, and I'm 14 lbs lighter!

Here's the bottom line: if you make the right decision, your body will thank you. You are what you eat – the food that goes in becomes your body's medicine. If you feed your body the wrong stuff it'll simply lay down fat whilst lowering your energy, sapping your sex drive and diminish your brain power.

By reading this chapter, you have the all-important first steps to a slimmer, healthier you. Good luck! Follow the "Kettlebell Fat Loss Blue Print" and watch how it changes your life.

"Jamie, what's the best workout for fat loss?" I can't tell you how many times I've heard that question in my career as a personal trainer. What I can tell you is that I've searched the world over looking for an answer, going to experts in the UK and the USA for their help.

The truth is there isn't one workout that's best for fat loss. If there was, it would be easy and everyone would look their best! There are, however, four common traits that show up in highly effective fat loss programs, and I'll tell you what they are.

STRENGTH TRAINING

Strength training increases lean tissue, which is metabolically active, burning calories even at rest. For fat loss, I typically recommend strength training in alternating supersets or a circuit. Why? Because when training opposite muscle groups, you can do a lot of work with just a little rest. This means a lot of calories burned over a short period of time – more bang for your buck!

HIGH-INTENSITY INTERVALS

A 1994 study by Tremblay suggested that alternating periods of very hard effort with periods of easy effort resulted in nine times more fat being burned than in steady-state endurance training. The interval group was tested over 15 weeks, compared to 20 weeks for the steady-state group. So high-intensity intervals help us burn nine times the fat in three quarters of the time.

EPOC

Short for "Excess Post-exercise Oxygen Consumption", EPOC comes as a result of hard training that creates a metabolic disturbance, elevating the metabolic rate for hours after the exercise session is over. This is related to both resistance training and intervals. It revs up the metabolism, causing greater calorie burn even at rest. Kettlebell training burns calories for around 24 hours after the workout. Compare this to a steady-state run, where you only burn calories for one or two hours afterwards.

CALORIE DEFICIT

Training hard and eating less will help you get lean. To create a calorie deficit, which will lead to fat loss, you have to work off more energy than the calories that you put in your mouth.

Now you know the four pillars for fat loss, let's get to work. I've put together three different plans and each one has two workouts. Do each one for four weeks and you'll have a complete 12-week fat loss training plan using only kettlebells.

THE KETTLEBELL FAT LOSS BLUEPRINT

Sunday ❑   Monday ❑   Tuesday ❑   Wednesday ❑   Thursday ❑   Friday ❑   Saturday ❑

Week One – 3 sets ❑ OFF ❑ Workout A ❑ OFF ❑ Workout B ❑ OFF ❑ Workout C ❑ OFF
Week Two – 3 sets ❑ OFF ❑ Workout C ❑ OFF ❑ Workout B ❑ OFF ❑ Workout A ❑ OFF
Week Three – 4 sets ❑ OFF ❑ Workout A ❑ OFF ❑ Workout C ❑ OFF ❑ Workout B ❑ OFF
Week Four – 4 sets ❑ OFF ❑ Workout C ❑ OFF ❑ Workout A ❑ OFF ❑ Workout B ❑ OFF

THE WORKOUTS

This program is based on doing three different workouts a week.

Workout A is a superset workout, using big bang exercises that utilize opposite muscles (for example a pushing exercise followed by a pulling exercise or a lower body exercise followed by an upper body exercise).

Workout B is a metabolic workout that will get your heart racing and give you an EPOC effect.

Workout C is a strength circuit that maximizes the 600 muscles in your body for maximum fat burning and overload.

When doing workout A, A1 & A2 are a super set. Do a set of A1, then A2, and then back to A1, until you have completed all the required sets. Then move on to the next pair of exercises.

Where the plan says 3-4 sets, try 3 for the first 2 weeks. You can always add another.

Tempo (rep speed) is expressed as a 3-digit number. The first number is the negative (or lowering), the second is pause, the third is the lifting (concentric). So a squat written as "311" would be a 3 second descent, 1 second pause and 1 second coming up. The 1 second lift is to be done as fast as possible.

A "quick" tempo applies to exercises that can't be done slowly, like snatches, or those that are done as fast as possible through the full range of motion.

Rest periods are written as "0" between exercises in a superset. If it says "1:00" that is the length between supersets or beginning the next exercise.

WORKOUT A

Exercise	Sets	Time	Tempo	Rest
A1 Front Squat Wide hand grip(KB)	3-4	30 secs	311	0
A2 Pushups off bells	3-4	30 secs	311	60 secs
B1 KB One Arm Bent Over Row	3-4	30 secs	321	0
B2 Clean & Press (tempo is pressing speed)	3-4	30 secs each side	311	60 secs
C1 Half Get Ups	3-4	5 reps each side	421	0
C2 Seated Russian Twists	3-4	30 secs	421	60 secs

WORKOUT B

Exercise	Time	Rest
Kettlebell 2 Arm Swings	30 secs	
Snatches	30 secs each arm	
Kettlebell 1 Arm Swings	30 secs each arm	
Clean, Squat and Press	30 secs each arm	
Kettlebell Alternate Arm Swings	30 secs	Rest for 1- 2minutes and repeat 5-6 rounds

For the timed workouts in A and B, do as many reps as you can safely complete in the given time. If you need to take a break, that's fine. If you can go the whole time without putting down the kettlebell, that is even better.

WORKOUT C

Exercise	Reps	Tempo	Rest
Full TGU	5 reps each	Quick	0
Renegade Rows	10 reps each	221	0
Tactical Lunges (KB)	10 reps each	321	0
Kettlebell High Pull	10 reps each	311	0
Double Front Squats	10 reps each	311	0
Double Military Presses	10	421	0
Windmills	5 reps each	321	0
Seated Hot Potato	30 secs	Fast paced	When you have completed the circuit, rest 1-2 minutes and repeat 3-4 rounds

Enjoy your Kettlebell Fat Loss Blueprint – and don't forget to stretch afterwards!

JAMIE'S TOP-TEN TIPS FOR RECLAIMING YOUR HEALTH

As we age, our blood ph-level becomes more acidic, attracting disease and accelerating the ageing process. An alkalising diet helps avoid this. Alkaline blood, which keeps the oxygen levels in our arteries higher and prevents the cells from degeneration, can only be achieved by consuming alkaline food and drinking alkaline water. Alkaline blood also prevents and can cure arthritis and gout. Uric acid (which causes the two ailments) can't be dissolved in water, alcohol or ether but does dissolve in alkaline salts and alkaline water.

Only alkaline blood can flush the toxins and wastes which are responsible for ageing out of the body. To maintain a high alkaline blood ph, at least 80% of our total food intake must comprise of alkaline foods.

In addition to the "Kettlebell Fat Loss Blue Print", try these simple steps to help slow down the ageing process.

TAKE ALKALISING SALTS

Sodium bicarbonate helps reduce the acidity in the muscles and blood. It also provides the body with a power boost to increase its endurance. Research also shows that taking sodium bi-carbonate reduces anxiety, helping manage the psychological affects of prolonged stress.

DRINK YOUR GREENS

Green drinks can make up for a lack of fruit and vegetables in our diets, helping prevent cancer, obesity and heart disease. Green drinks containing grasses like wheat grass, barley grass and alfalfa, sprouted grains and green vegetables give your body easily-absorbed vitamins, minerals and amino acids.

DRINK FILTERED WATER

Drinking filtered water reduces chlorine and chlorine compounds as well as other undesirables from tap water like heavy metals (including lead and copper) caused by household plumbing pipes.

BE ASLEEP BY 10:30PM

Late nights cause our bodies to release cortisol, a stress hormone, which contributes to weight-gain. Elevated cortisol levels are associated with increase cravings and appetite, extra body fat, decreased muscle mass and bone density, increased anxiety and depression and reduced libido. Mood-swings, memory impairment and increased PMS symptoms are also likely effects.

EAT 75% RAW ORGANIC FOOD

Try eating 75% raw food rather than processed foods. Heating food above 118*F destroys enzymes that assist in digestion and absorption. Go for organic uncooked plant foods such as fresh fruit and vegetables, sprouts, seeds, nuts, grains, beans, dried fruit and seaweed.

VITAMIN D

A vitamin D supplement will improve your immune system and is essential for absorbing calcium and phosphorous (for bone and tooth growth). A lack of vitamin D has been linked to cravings for carbs and sugary foods.

MAGNESIUM

Magnesium deficiency has been linked to diabetes, heart disease and osteoporosis. Magnesium helps open up the cells to bring in nutrients.

SELENIUM WITH IODINE

Selenium and iodine are critically important in the proper functioning of the thyroid. Taking both will help detox the body and get rid of chlorine, fluorides and other toxins which compromise thyroid function, cellular metabolism and hormonal balance.

VITAMIN C

Humans are unable to synthesize vitamin C, and it therefore must be attained from our diets or a supplement. Vitamin C is vital for the formation and maintenance of connective tissue, amino acid metabolism and protection from chemicals.

LECITHIN

Lecithin can be found in the major organs of the heart, the liver, and the kidneys and is used by every cell in our bodies. Although it's found in many common foods, the average diet just doesn't supply enough of it. Lecithin supplementation is necessary for overall health and prevention of many conditions and diseases.

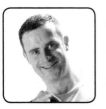

ABOUT JAMIE

Jamie Lloyd has been at the forefront of the UK health and fitness industry for over eight years and holds certifications from some of the most prestigious personal training, sports medicine and therapy academies around the world. His knowledge and experience as a strength and Kettlebell coach is combined with over 25 years of intensive physical training in rugby union, martial arts, football, long distance running, duathlons and triathlons.

One of only a handful of elite Russian Kettlebell Coaches in Europe, Jamie is a certified Russian Kettlebell Challenge (RKC) Instructor and is an IKFF (International Kettlebell Fitness Federation) Level 2 Kettlebell Coach which is also recognised as a world-class Kettlebell qualification. He is also an assistant to Steve Cotter at the IKFF team. He has developed his very own KettleFIT System TM, Joint Mobility Manual TM, Kettlebell Concepts Manual TM, Kettlebell Concepts Course TM, KettleFIT Classes TM and Detoxification Diet TM, in which all have helped hundreds of people improve their movement of dysfunction, biochemistry and nutrition to create what is arguably some of the most complete health promotion systems available today.

Seen as one of the UK's top fitness experts Jamie has become renowned for being an inspirational teacher of Kettlebells, and is the director of Russian Kettlebells UK. Through his passion for fitness he has helped hundreds of personal trainers, sports therapists, physios, osteopaths and athletes become proficient in the use of Kettlebells and his KettleFIT system TM.

Jamie's multi-disciplinary approach has attracted clients from all walks of life and all backgrounds including elite level athletes, martial artists and medical backgrounds. He has also been seen in Mens Fitness and Mens Health Magazine and a number of national newspapers. He also writes regularly for US Kettlebell Sport and Fitness magazine called http://kettlebellmag.com and also for a UK Kettlebell Magazine called http://www.kettlebell-fit.com

Whilst devoting his time and energy to his one-to-one clients he still manages to work full time as a Firefighter for the London Fire Brigade.

If you would like to book Jamie for personal training, kettlebell classes, or a kettlebell training course, or if you are a member of the press with a query, then please contact Jamie at jamie@russiankettlebellsuk.com or visit http://www.russiankettlebellsuk.com

CHAPTER 5

NOT YOUR TYPICAL 'FAT KID TO FITNESS PHENOMENON' STORY

BY BEN WARSTLER

My story starts out in a pretty typical manner. I grew up overweight and was teased relentlessly by kids, …at school, on the bus, and just plain 'out in public'. I had very low self-esteem and a firm belief that I was always going to be overweight and a constant 'punching bag' for those who were 'better than me'.

With low self-esteem, I always fidgeted with my clothes because I was uncomfortable in them and never took my shirt off in public – all the things that a 'fat kid' experiences in their childhood. I was however, athletic, and enjoyed playing sports very much. I found it was an outlet for my frustration with my body and more importantly, for my mind. This would later fail me, but more on that in a bit. When I wasn't playing sports, I was thinking about playing, because if I didn't, I thought about myself, and if I could avoid that, I would at all costs.

Now that doesn't sound much different to most 'fat kid' stories you have heard in the past, so you're probably wondering what the heck I have to offer that is so different to every other 'fat kid transformation' story you have ever heard. Well I'll tell you in a minute, but first I want to give you a little background as to where I am now compared to where I was. I'm going to refer to my business because my business is my outlet now for all the frustrations, and serves as a bit of a payback to all those naysayers that have ever encountered me in my life.

So to give you a quick rundown: I run fitness bootcamps. And not only do I run them, I run them well. It's the main source of income in my life. I currently have over 215 bootcamp clients. Now there are other bootcamp businesses that are that large, and perhaps larger. However, what sets my business apart from all others is the size of the client base I'm pulling from. I live in Northeast Vermont, an area called the Northeast Kingdom and the largest town in our area is 5,000 people. I have two locations each with 100 campers per town. But it's truly not the numbers that I'm most proud of. Each of our locations has a Wall of Fame for those who have changed their lives. They are a sampling of what our program has been able to do for people. For every plaque that is on each wall, there are three to four others that have had their lives changed through our program. I could easily talk about my clients all day and their successes, but that's not what is going to help you the most.

Let me get back to my story. After high school, I no longer played organized sports so I would play intramurals in college and that is when I discovered the 'weight room'. I learned 'on the fly' by watching others workout. I emulated what they did. Some things worked well, and others I will never do again. It was amazing how many different things people did in the gym. I had found my new outlet and I practiced it religiously, almost to the point of obsession. I put it into my regular schedule immediately. What I didn't realize at the time is that not only had I found an outlet, but I had also found a passion. And it wasn't just the transformation I was undergoing, and it wasn't even the exercise itself that I had developed a passion for, …it was the escape. I was able to escape my thoughts, feelings, and emotions that tormented me the entire time I wasn't in the gym. What I also gained an appreciation of was for the people that were also making changes, by taking the time to be conscious about their looks and or health. However, those very same people also served as motivation – almost to the point of competition for me. You see, the competitive spirit I developed as an athlete followed me into this life! I had to be better than they were, so the rivalry of me vs. everyone else was born. It was this very moment that set the stage for where I am today, both physically and in business.

Everyone was a competitor to me, at least when I was in the gym. I had to outwork everyone there, …to lift more and push out more reps than anyone else. I channeled the motivation I always had in sports to my health and self-improvement. In the meantime, *I was also changing my mindset.*

Just a side note here, when I refer to mindset, I'm not referring to eliminating the 'fat kid' mentality, because I firmly believe that never goes away. Once a 'fat kid' always a 'fat kid'. A 'fat kid' will always have a less than positive feeling about how they look and how they are portrayed by others, no matter how much success is reached. I know this from firsthand experience, but I also know others who carry the 'fat kid' on their back, despite all the success physically and financially they may have achieved. It is crystal clear to me that money and good looks will not give you happiness if your mind still believes you are poor and unattractive. What I'm referring to when I say mindset is that I was changing how I would approach every day, and in all actuality used the 'fat kid' talk in my head to motivate me in my physical outlet. I was competing against everyone to be better than they were, but what I was really competing against was myself, and the 'good' me was winning.

I developed a mentality when I trained where I'm not social at all, and it was to the point that I was actually mean when I was training. It was all because I had conditioned my brain to be in a specific state that accepted nothing but my best effort every single time. And every time, I would train myself to exhaustion mentally and/or physically, so by the time I left the gym, I had returned to my 'so called normal' mental state.

FAST FORWARD TO TODAY

Over the years I have been able to harness this mentality to allow it to carry over to my business and my life. I credit almost all of my business success to training my mind to compete with everyone around me who either pose a threat or have something less than kind to say (fat kids are also sensitive). I don't know how many times I was told I wouldn't be able to do it or someone had the mannerisms that showed I was just a 'flash in the pan'. It was those very actions or words that fueled a fire within me that has brought me to where I am today, and which will take me to where I want to go in the future.

It is these very characteristics that I try to pass on to my clients so that they can be successful. However, despite my best attempts to pass them on, I have discovered a very sobering fact: most people will not be successful in their attempts. They are too busy looking for the next great exercise or super food that is going to save them and carry them 'to the promised land' of being happy about how they look and feel. Well, I'm here to tell you that there is no super food, no magic pill or exercise routine that is going to give you what you want if your mind isn't on board. So how the heck do you do that? Ultimately, only you will know what drives you, what fuels your undying, killer instinct to keep eating supportively, to not miss a workout, and to just plain 'keep your head down and go full steam ahead.' I can't help you with what motivates you. I can ask questions such as, 'What will happen if you don't take action?' Your answer to that question will often tell the story as to 'how bad you want it'. Now, while I can't tell you how to answer that question, and I cannot motivate you, I can direct you to steps you can take to create the mindset that will best prepare you to take your mind and body to the next level.

FIVE STEPS TO TRAIN YOUR MIND FOR A TOTAL BODY BREAKTHROUGH

1. The first and most important step is to write down what you want to achieve. Thinking about it is one thing, but there is something to be said about writing it down. Use as much detail as you can, so that you are painting a picture on paper that is in your mind. It often helps to write it down in paragraph form, sort of like an affirmation. Write it down in the present tense as if it has already happened. A quick story of the success of this approach: a couple years ago I participated in a goal-setting program designed to accomplish more than I ever had before. I started the program, wrote down and prioritized what I wanted to accomplish. I lost track over time of the list but just came across it about a month ago. To my astonishment 75% of the goals had been accomplished and I had completely forgotten I had wrote them down. The 'kicker' here is that these goals were a mix of everyday habit changes and big goals that, before

writing them down, I didn't fully believe I would ever achieve them.

Needless to say, write your goals down and read them every day.

2. Now that you have your goals written down and you are reading them daily, its time to take action. It may sound obvious that this is the next step but many people don't get beyond writing down their goals. They believe that writing them down will automatically make it happen. But if I wrote down that I want a million dollars, that doesn't put the million in my pocket. In terms of training your mind, its important to start small with taking action. Don't expect to make landmark changes overnight, you will become overwhelmed way too soon. However, once you get comfortable with the changes you have made, don't be afraid to get a little aggressive. Now you're probably asking yourself, 'this chapter was about training your mind, and now you're talking about goals?' What gives?' By setting small, very simple goals you are training your subconscious mind, and training your mind to become positive on a more regular basis. You can certainly change your 'self talk' from negative to positive but that's easier said than done, and quite frankly I see that advice as being a bit of a 'cop out'. You can't just suddenly change how you talk to yourself. Setting small simple habit-changing goals and accomplishing them will go a long way to changing how you talk about yourself.

3. Remember where you were, and constantly revisit how you felt. It may sound counterproductive, but it has helped me more times than I can count. Its no secret that you will have peaks and valleys with your motivation and success. The obvious goal is to minimize those valleys as much as possible, so that you can be consistent with your success. When I'm in a rut and stuck with inconsistency, it often is because of rationalization. Rationalizations are justifications we all use to validate our excuses, …to fall off track with nutrition, exercise, or anything that has to do with your goals. Eliminating rationalizations is a tremendous undertaking and may not be necessary.

What I'm referring to by remembering where you were and to

revisit how you felt, just means it helps me tremendously to remember how down on myself I used to feel – before I started taking action to make changes. It helps me remember where I am going and where I never want to return. It allows me to refuel my motivation and to keep going. (I see it as moving further and further away from where I was, so continuing to challenge myself to improve moves me towards a goal; but for me, more importantly, away from where I never want to be again.)

4. Realize that you are one of the select few. Realizing that you are one of the select few that is really making legitimate changes will go a long way toward transforming your efforts inside and out. Think this is a little conceited? Well perhaps it is, but when was the last time you thought positive thoughts of yourself? This is all part of the transformation, so if you are struggling with this step, you may not be ready for it. What I suggest is to continue setting and achieving small goals. This is a very important step because it will protect you against difficult times where you will want to 'forget it all' and revert right back to your old habits. You are expanding your comfort zone and 'stepping out of your box'; you better be proud of yourself and you better understand that 99% of the world's population will never experience stepping outside their comfort zone. Once you realize this fact, the possibilities are endless.

5. Share your success with others. Your last step is to spread your success. Sharing your success allows you to continue your motivation and enhance your positivity about yourself. You are able to achieve more and being recognized is always a tremendous motivator to continue your success. The thought that enters my mind when I first encounter a new client is that they are probably feeling the same way if not worse than I did at my lowest point. I feel compelled to share with them the tools so that they can be successful. I'm not asking you to become a trainer or coach at all. What I am asking is for you to share with others the tools you have learned, so you might be able to help someone else feel better about themselves, and in turn you will feel more confident about yourself. There is nothing quite like

helping someone with the tools you have used to be successful, so that they too may be successful.

Every single one of these steps I still practice and use daily. It is vital to understand that these changes are not temporary. Settle in, because these are tools you will take with you forever. Practice, master, and re-peat over–and-over and over–and-over again. However, once you have accomplished these tasks and are consistent with your efforts, they will become habits and you will have changed your mindset to attack and conquer your goals, …and anything will be possible!

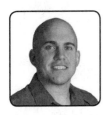

ABOUT BEN

Ben Warstler, CSCS, NSCA-CPT, KBA is the owner of Bens Boot-camps in Northeast Vermont. Growing his business from 8 boot camp clients to over 200 in less than three years in two towns of less than 4000 people, Ben is one of the world's most successful boot camp business owners. Ben is currently a coach with the best boot camp business coaching program on the market today, The Bootcamp Blueprint. Ben is also the creator of Bens Bootcamps Home Fat Loss System, and has spoken at national seminars and workshops.

Ben Warstler, CSCS, NSCA-CPT

The Bootcamp Emperor

Groundbreaking Fitness, LLC

www.bensbootcamps.com

www.vermontbootcamps.com

http://benwarstler.com

CHAPTER 6

A FRESH NUTRITION PARADIGM

BY JON LE TOCQ

N utrition is without doubt the most misunderstood and perhaps, the most underrated element of health and fitness training.

Many of those keen to make serious improvement to their body composition, physique and strength now appear to recognise that a great training program will yield little without excellent nutrition habits. However, it is clear from the prevalence of sickness, lethargy and poor recovery from intense exercise that the focus is misdirected.

Recent years have seen the rapid growth in popularity of high protein, low fat, low carb diets as the way to build lean muscle and keep body fat to a minimum.

However, a different school of thought is gaining momentum as the focus shifts to targeting health and performance, whilst still creating lean, muscular physiques.

What follows is based not only on review of scientific literature, but also anecdotal experience with family, friends and clients.

The key questions that should be asked in all cases of chasing a health, fitness or performance target are simple, but rarely answered with clear vision.

*'What will this do **for** me and **to** me?'*

For instance, there is no doubt that a high protein diet combined with a high volume training program, will lead to a significant increase in lean muscle. The program will give you a more muscular physique.

But in terms of what it will do **to** you, we need to dig deeper.

In today's world, most meat which doesn't 'cost the earth', is full of steroids and antibiotics. As usual profits drive actions. Many animals bred for meat are fast-tracked through the growth process using growth hormone and steroid chemicals – in order to fatten them up in their cramped living conditions ready for slaughter.

Not only does this lead to higher levels of saturated fat due to lack of exercise, but it also means that the lucky consumer now gets to ingest a steak full of steroids.

Some herds are then indiscriminately given antibiotics to combat mastitis and other illnesses – which could reduce profits. Done routinely, this helps antibiotic-resistant bacteria to dominate, which then end up in your food and in your gut. Why does this matter if all you want is big muscles?

If your intestine is full of antibiotic-resistant bacteria, your digestive system will soon run into difficulty. This means less energy assimilated from food leading to substandard training, as well as fewer nutrients absorbed to aid the digestion and use of protein in the body. Ultimately this means impaired muscle recovery and growth. This will put the brakes on even the best training programs in the long run!

The highly acidic nature of animal protein also means you are setting yourself up for poor health and chronic systemic inflammation which is likely to manifest eventually as sore muscles after training, ill health, chronic aches and pains and increased risk of metabolic and cardiovascular disease.

It is therefore my belief that for optimal, long-term muscle growth and performance gains, high protein diets must be used in short, intermittent bursts if at all.

I personally choose a largely vegetarian nutrition approach, but if you choose to have high protein periods, ensure they are interspersed with periods of low animal protein intake accompanied by very high levels of raw foods to restore the function of the digestive system.

The animal protein you do consume should consist of organic, grass-fed beef wherever possible, seawater fish, organic, free-range eggs and a range of plant foods containing varying amounts of the amino acids required for lean muscle growth.

Look at the long-term health and performance benefits. Are 3 months of 'amazing' muscle growth worth the risk of training and sports performance dropping, and ill health, when a muscular, athletic physique can be gained somewhat more slowly but with much longer-lasting and impressive results?

The concept of macronutrient cycling or flexing can and should be applied on a month-to-month basis as well as day-to-day and even hourly.

Carbohydrates are another grossly misunderstood macronutrient. We are currently in the low carb era in which we are led to believe that simply looking at a carbohydrate-based food will make you fat! Again the reality lies in a question.

"What do I need, why do I need it and when?"

Not only do high performance athletes and 'weekend warriors' need carbohydrates for energy in order to train hard, but carbohydrates are also a critical element of the muscle building process, putting you in an anabolic state.

Chronic carb **deprivation** will lead to stagnant results, static body composition and constant bad moods and irritability.

Chronic high carb **intake** will lead to high body fat levels and likely the onset of diabetic conditions due to insulin resistance.

The trick again is 'flexing' your carb intake.

After intense exercise, whether it be metabolic conditioning or high volume weight training, the body is at its peak of insulin sensitivity. This means that carbohydrate consumption at this time will result in refuelling of depleted muscle glycogen ready for the next bout, and fuel for the energy-intensive activity that is muscle growth. It will also play a critical part in the anabolic processes that follow weight training.

You need not worry about conversion to body fat if you have worked yourself hard!

Carbohydrates can be ingested in pure powder form (e.g basic maltodextrin or Vitargo) in post workout shakes along with your protein of choice. Whilst short periods of whey consumption may not cause any unwanted side-effects, long-term I would focus on rice and pea protein and hemp protein options.

A ratio of 4:1 carbohydrates to protein with 1g of carbohydrates for each kilogram of bodyweight for every hour you trained, will serve you well as a post-training shake. So if you weigh 100kg you would have 100g of maltodextrin or Vitargo with 25g of protein.

I would also add Branch Chain Amino Acids before and after weight training for more intense sessions and better anabolic effects. Alternatively, use this post-training window to take in fruits in your shake so that you also get the bonus of antioxidants in your recovery drink.

If you find this not to be enough, you should then consider more carbs in your post-workout meal. Rice or sweet potatoes would be a great option. At all other times, carbohydrate intake should be low in order to avoid gains in body fat or chronic insulin secretion, which can lead to insulin resistance in the long-term.

If you are a naturally skinny person struggling to gain muscle, you should increase your intake of fats from sources such as olive oil, coconut oil, flax seed oil, avocados, nuts and oily fish, rather than gorging on carbs.

Even on a muscle building effort, I would recommend one low calorie day per week or per fortnight, in order to allow the digestive muscles a rest from the high calorie intake. This may also lead to a boost in growth hormone.

Digestive muscles need rest and recovery in the same way your 'showcase' muscles do!

Now we need to take a step back from the details of macronutrient cycling and make sure you have the basics in place!

Let's start with a quick fire round on water, as very, very few people are sufficiently hydrated to function properly on a basic level, never-mind engage in high intensity training and chase performance objectives! Whole books have been written on the importance of water but I am going to cherry pick areas directly related to your training performance.

First, water is what gives structure to your intervertebral discs. Given that 75% of your upper body weight is supported by water volume in these discs, dehydration will lead to smaller 'cushions' thus greatly increasing your risk of low back pain.

This applies to 'Average Joe'.

Add some heavy back squats, deadlifts, kettlebell swings or simply hard running to your dehydrated state, and you can expect issues at your 5th lumbar vertebra, waving goodbye to the intense training sessions that bring great results!

Similarly, dehydration will lead to poor joint cartilage structure increasing your risk of rheumatoid arthritis and cutting short your 'training life' as joint remodelling takes hold from all the abuse in training and competition.

Never walk into a training session with a dry mouth. By then, adequate hydration levels are long gone. From a bodyweight perspective, sensations of thirst and hunger go hand-in-hand as the brain demands energy for function.

Unfortunately, most people reach for the food first, so being chronically dehydrated can leave you believing you are permanently hungry and in need of sugars. This leads to a vicious cycle of snacking, overeating and not dealing with the root cause.

If you are strong enough to ignore the 'hunger' sensations to stay on track for low body fat, that's great, but not rehydrating your body will still leave it in survival or storage mode.

In this state your body is getting concerned about lack of nutrients and will start to store anything and everything for energy reserves. You can forget any energy being used for unnecessary activities like muscle building. Your body doesn't know that the fridge and water fountain are around the corner and so will start switching off anything that doesn't aid life preservation.

Finally, brain function is heavily dependant on energy formed from water as well as glucose – just like all other muscles.

During periods of mental stress such as a demanding time at work, energy requirements in the brain increase. If insufficient water is available for the production of 'hydroenergy', your body will ask for the next best thing – more sugar.

This is when the cravings start!

The body is designed for long periods of low intensity movement that are now non-existent in most peoples' desk-bound jobs. This kind of movement stimulates the hormone lipase that aids fat breakdown for fuel. Without the stimulation of lipase, blood sugar must be used up, leaving less available for brain function. The cravings that follow can be devastating.

Be aware that sodas such as Diet Coke and other caffeine rich drinks are a very bad option when mentally stressed. The caffeine and aspartame contained in them are potent neurotransmitter exciters. This will only lead to greater blood sugar usage and cravings for refuelling.

Finally, a word on raw food.

Raw food, behind water, is probably the most important feature on any nutrition plan.

Not only do raw, uncooked vegetables contain a high level of minerals and fibre, but they also provide the digestive enzymes that will enable you to better absorb the minerals and energy from your food.

More energy and minerals such as iron, calcium and magnesium means better bone strength and muscle building potential.

Green vegetables and grasses offer very high levels of chlorophyll – which is effectively the 'blood' of plants, thus bringing high levels of energy into your own body. It also reduces binding of carcinogens to cells in the liver, so hugely important for long-term health.

Greens drinks containing alfalfa grass, barley grass and wheat grass are potent sources of chlorophyll and can lead to instant increases in energy and vitality, whether you're a beginner or an elite athlete.

Wheat grass contains every identified mineral and trace mineral, including higher levels of iron than spinach as well as every vitamin in the B complex – crucial for energy conversion and a high metabolic rate.

Barley grass has 3 times more Vitamin C than spinach and 7 times more than oranges. Daily intake will lead to higher levels of stamina, sexual energy and thought clarity, and reduced addictions to healthy food.

The combination promises more intense training, greater productivity at work, faster fat loss and more fun!

Alfalfa grass is great for improving the function of your digestive tract and kidneys.

This is crucial, especially if you're consuming a high protein diet which can put strain on the kidneys. When the kidneys are under pressure the liver takes over some of the workload, meaning it has less 'availability' for one of its primary functions – fat metabolism.

If your liver isn't functioning properly, you're putting the brakes on potential fat loss, so up your greens in the form of vegetables and daily greens drinks.

So, rather than rehashing the usual 'physique transformation' nutrition advice, it is my belief that a paradigm shift is necessary. Implementing the key principles in this chapter will enable you to shift your mindset to one of targeting health and physical performance.

This is vital if you are to live a healthy fitness lifestyle full of intense training, competition on the sports field and of course, develop a lean, muscular physique.

A simple change of focus will reap incredible rewards for the rest of your life, not just on the beach this summer!

There is no need for a trade-off between looking great and optimizing your health, energy and physical performance.

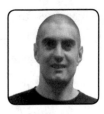

ABOUT JON

Jon Le Tocq is a leading British health and performance coach. Having worked with a wide range of clients – from elite athletes to stressed out business people, he has developed cutting-edge nutrition and training strategies to restore health and optimize physical performance both day-to-day and on the sports field.

Find out more at: www.stormforcefitness.com

CHAPTER 7

SECRETS TO STAYING ON TRACK DURING WEIGHT LOSS

BY KIM CHASE

Trying to stay on track and follow all the rules, while trying to lose weight and reach new goals, can be the most challenging aspect of weight loss. I've seen some of my strongest clients (with regards to will power), veer off track and plummet because of a bad day that led to cheating and bingeing. Then comes the guilt for doing it and wondering if it's ever going to happen for you; if you'll ever reach your goals and be that slim, toned person you so desire to be.

All is not lost. One must be persistent and diligent in your quest and don't let small obstacles sabotage your efforts. Yea, sure it's going to be tough, you're going to have your pitfalls and your stumbling blocks, but the biggest thing is not to lose sight of your end goal and believe that it can and will be achieved. It's either persevere and win your war, or give up, slip into depression, hate your body and continuously stay where you hate being…fat.

I'll share a little story with you. After I had my two boys, I blossomed and gained 45 lbs over my pre-pregnancy weight. I stayed there for about 3 years wishing and wondering if I was ever going to get rid of this unsightly fat that surrounded my slim physique underneath. I had always been athletic, I was a competitive gymnast, later a body builder, equestrian jumper, and played just about every other sport I could get into. I hated the way I looked and couldn't stand the fact that I let myself get this way. But I kept blaming it on the baby fat, it was my excuse. When was it going to be enough already! I needed to stop making excuses.

It wasn't until I started to build my own house that I got back into physical activity. Hauling lumber and breaking down walls takes a lot of energy! I started to see changes in my shape and size and then started to feel better; I actually got excited about fitness again. I became more aware of what I was eating and made every day a workout. Since I spent most of my day at the house, I purposely took a task and made it a workout since making time for the gym was not an option. I needed to find this different avenue of exercise because I dreaded going back to the gym knowing it was going to take a lot of effort. For six months I toiled away at building, lifting, hauling and every functional movement possible with huge efforts and ate properly. Before I knew it I was down 8 sizes and 45 pounds. I loved it and it felt great again. My point is, find something you like doing in order to find fitness again. Make it a purposeful workout and start to feel good again. You'll find that getting to the gym after that is much easier and a much more welcome venture – you'll even look forward to it.

I've compiled a check list of all the things to do or not to do while you're trying to lose weight. Everything you need to know to help you stay on track. "Your perseverance will turn into a habit, and that habit will turn into a lifestyle."

1. Never lose sight of your goals – the minute you lose focus on your end goals is the minute you start to slip back to where you started. Stay focused, and don't ever forget what direction you're heading in. If you slip, get right back on it.

2. Keep a positive attitude, believe in yourself – The "I can do this" attitude is critical to your success. You need to tell yourself that this is doable, no second guessing – ever! You are a great person and worth the effort.

3. Set goals – don't just focus on the long term goal, you'll get frustrated and lose your motivation. Keep your goals small and obtainable. Set weekly goals, like – 'I'm going to lose 3 pounds this week,' and monthly goals, like increasing your reps or weight load during exercise. This will give you the results you seek and keep you motivated.

4. Don't live by the scale! Take your measurements weekly and track your losses that way. Some weeks you'll only lose a pound or even less, but inches will be coming off. Our bodies exchange adipose (fat) tissue for lean muscle mass. Muscle weighs two times more than fat and fat tissue has 20% more volume. Once you can comprehend that fact, you'll be able to let go of the scale and rely on your clothing size. Use the scale at the end of your weight loss when you can keep track of where you need to remain. It is only a guide to let you know if you've slipped from your target weight and body composition.

5. Get rid of temptation – clean house! Get rid of everything bad in your cupboards. No sweets, chips, alcohol, processed or canned foods. They all have added salt or sugar or chemical preservatives that will hinder healthy eating.

6. Be Rid Of Boredom! – get busy, find hobbies, get outside in the evening, (which is the worst time for snackers), take the dog for a walk or walk with a friend, and don't sit in front of the TV. Boredom breeds eating!

7. Don't beat yourself up – when you slip up, acknowledge it, stop it, and move on. If you dwell on it you will only continue to eat, and the wrong things at that, guaranteed. It's better to stop where you're at and get back on track, than it is to keep depressing yourself because you screwed up, which results in more eating.

8. Tell someone weekly what your short term goals are, it makes you more accountable.

9. The 'this time' rule – I got this one from a client of mine and I love it. Always ask yourself what are you going to do 'this time'? Are you going to eat that cookie or are you going to grab

an apple 'this time'? Are you going to take the elevator, or are you going to take the stairs 'this time'? Are you going to sit in front of the TV tonight, or are you going take a walk 'this time'? You get the picture. Make yourself the judge and jury.

10. Find support – if your family doesn't support your journey (and believe it or not, some don't, they don't want you to leave them behind fat, so they sabotage your goals), then find friends or a support group that you can turn to.

11. Set the example – your kids follow your lead. By letting them eat all the bad foods that you do not only sets them up for obesity and high health risks, but you are also giving them permission to be that way. You have given them your blessing to get fat and unhealthy; and we're supposed to protect and nurture our children.

   Okay, that was all the psychological stuff you need to work on, now here's the nutritional and fitness stuff that's going to make you or break you. So listen up.

12. Lots of water! – drink ½ your body weight in ounces daily. So if you weigh 200 lbs, you need to drink 100 ounces of water every day. Water flushes out toxins from the body, keeps you hydrated, especially for those wicked workouts you have planned, and keeps your body functioning in many ways.

13. Eat within 1 hour of waking – This is really important, your body needs to know it can stop fasting and get the metabolism working first thing. If you haven't triggered your metabolism with that wake up call, it still thinks it's in storage mode and it won't let go of any of the fat deposits to use for energy. Instead it will attack the amino acids (muscle tissue) in your body and use that for its energy source. The last thing you want to do is start eliminating your muscle tissue.

14. Eat every 2 – 3 hours throughout the day. Again, you have a window to feed the body before it goes into storage mode, and if you don't trigger your metabolism to break down food, then it automatically stores what it had before as fat and then targets the muscles for its energy source. So in the end, all you are is weak and fat.

15. Try not to eat 2 – 3 hours before sleeping. You want the body to go to sleep in the fat burning mode. If you eat before sleeping, most likely it contains a carb of some sort, whether it is simple or complex. The body will automatically use the carbs for its energy source and burn off what you ate instead of what you already have stored. Therefore, your body will be in a carb burning state during rest instead of the desired fat burning state.

16. Eat Carbs early – simple and starchy carbs should be eaten during the earlier parts of your day so you can burn them off. By consuming them early on in the day, by mid afternoon at the latest, the body will use them for its primary energy source instead of storing them as fat, especially when our bodies start to slow down for the evening. Starchy carbs should be whole wheat or whole grains, and select sweet potatoes over white, and brown or wild rice over white. Here's a good rule of thumb, "if it's white, out of sight".

17. Eat protein with every meal. Don't skip on this one! Protein gives your body the building blocks to support lean muscle mass. Lean muscle mass jacks up your metabolism and burns calories. Without protein, you have nothing to replenish your muscles with, so they deteriorate and build layers of flab on them. Women especially tend to forget about protein with their meals, and it has been reported that as soon as they start adding proper amounts of protein to their diet, they begin losing weight, even without trying.

18. Use smaller plates and bowls – don't use the standard dinner size plates, use the salad plate size or a kids plate, and use dessert bowls instead of soup bowls. This will keep your portions in check and trick the mind that you're getting a larger serving. Don't go for seconds unless it's veggies and salad.

19. Portion control – here's an easy way to gauge your portions without having to measure: ½ of your plate should be salad, ¼ of your plate should be another vegetable or a healthy starchy carb (nothing white), and ¼ of your plate protein.

20. Journal your food intake – if you write it down, you can track

what you are doing, right or wrong. It makes you accountable and very aware of what you're putting in your body. It's amazing how many people I've come across that were shocked how they ate because they simply became aware of it.

21. Do resistance training – whether it is with weights, bands or simple body weight, it is essential to have it in your fitness routine. Remember, you must have lean muscle mass to burn calories efficiently. Resistance training improves metabolism, circulation, flexibility, muscle tone, builds muscular endurance and strength, reduces stress and tension, reduces the risk of injuries, increases bone density, improves core strength and posture, increases tendon and ligament strength, and reduces the loss of lean muscle mass due to aging and inactivity.

22. Do cardiovascular training – include cardio training in any conditioning or weight loss program, it is absolutely necessary for good heart health; and it makes daily life a whole lot easier. It's going to decrease body fat, increase heart efficiency, lower blood pressure and cholesterol, lower risk of heart disease, lower resting heart rate, increase blood volume and capillary density, increase lung capacity and cardio-endurance.

23. Form is everything – whenever doing any fitness program, keep a good grip on your form. The minute you lose proper form, you lose the exercise; if you lose the exercise, you lose the purpose.

24. Look for fun things to do with the family as an alternative to a workout. Take them hiking for the afternoon, or go for a family bike ride, get a baseball game going with some neighborhood kids. When was the last time you played tag, now that's a great cardio workout! Take them to a public pool and keep up with them! Whew! If you have a dog, make sure you get him out for a brisk walk or jog daily, and get the kids out so it's a family event. It not only gets them active but teaches them that our pets need to be active too.

25. Work place tips:

   i.   Always take the stairs, and if you don't have bad knees or hips, take two at a time.

ii. Use the bathroom which is farthest away.

iii. Walk over to a co-worker instead of emailing them.

iv. Every ½ hour walk around the office, keep your legs and arms moving to keep circulation peaked and reduce stiffness.

v. Go for a brisk walk at lunch time instead of heading to the restaurant with co-workers, then come back and eat. You will not only ignite the fat burning mode, but you will then replenish your body with needed proteins and complex carbs.

vi. Stand up and move around every time you take a drink of water.

vii. Stand and/or walk around the room when talking on the phone.

viii. Take a 5 minute walk break with every coffee break.

26. Reward yourself – this is a big one. Don't let your successes go unnoticed; reward yourself every time you meet a new goal. Take yourself out to a movie, get a pedicure, buy yourself a new pair of shoes or some great runners, get a barber shave with a facial. Whatever floats your boat to make you feel special, go do it when you achieve a new level. But whatever you do, never reward yourself with food. We don't want to fire up any old habits.

So there you have it, everything you need to know to help you make it to your end goals. If you commit and follow these rules, success will be yours, I promise you. Learn to "eat to live and not live to eat." Take pride in the fact that you are making changes to live a long, healthy life. You are worth every bit of the effort!

ABOUT KIM

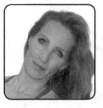

Kim Chase, CPTS, of Chase Fitness in Thunder Bay, Ontario, Canada has been involved in fitness her whole life. With experience in varied athletics such as competitive gymnastics, body building, soccer and baseball, equestrian jumping, skiing, Tae Kwon Do and anything else that looked like fun at the moment, Kim has harnessed that energy and passion to help others reach their own physical and mental goals.

Kim spent 10 years in the military, 6 years as an F-18 aircraft mechanic and 4 years as a pilot. In her off time she put her time in at the local fire hall as a firefighter which she continued with in the different locations she resided in. She spent 3 years up the Arctic in Iqaluit, on Baffin Island where she was the first female Chief Inspector for the Nunavut Liquor Commission. After moving back to Thunder Bay, her home town, she became certified in personal training where she worked in a local club. Kim is now an independent personal trainer building her own business. She specializes in weight loss, strength training and corrective mobility. All this is accomplished through one-on-one training, semi-private training, public boot camps and corporate wellness programs.

Her main focus is to get people motivated, strong, eating right and moving functionally through joint and tissue mobility and stability. This equates to healthy living, weight loss and disease reduction. It's important for her to make her clients understand that a healthy lifestyle will keep them living longer and functioning smoothly into their golden years. So educating them is part of the process of a healthy lifestyle; "I don't sugar coat things, this is what's going to happen to you if you continue down this path", she says. "People need to hear it like it is or they just don't get it. Too many of us have people around us using the soft approach about our health and don't want to make waves. Well, that doesn't work! Bottom line is that if you are not determined to eat right and exercise, your health will be determined for you – and it's not a positive outlook."

Her first-hand experience as a cancer survivor, twice through, has allowed Kim to relate to and deal with people in the same circumstances, knowing that a certain level of fitness is mandatory for expedited recovery and prevention.

Kim is certified through Can-Fit Pro as a Personal Trainer and is also a Certified Coach of The Canadian Gymnastics Federation, and Certified Judging Official in Gymnastics and Track and Field. She has earned herself a gold and silver medal in Tae Kwon Do at the Can Am Games.

Kim believes that inside every person is a dynamic individual that can achieve anything they want – when they set their mind to it.

"The mind leads the body, so just tell it to move!"

CHAPTER 8

MENTAL TOUGHNESS: THE KEY TO YOUR FITNESS SUCCESS

BY PAT RIGSBY

When it comes to achieving fitness or physical performance goals there are dozens, no, make that hundreds of different approaches that you can take to reach your desired destination. Low carb, low fat, South Beach, Weight Watchers, Jenny Craig and NutriSystem each can display plenty of success stories and that's just a few of the approaches to dieting. Exercise is the same. Pick any exercise system and it will have its share of true believers and glowing testimonials.

Well, I'd be lying to you if I told you that I thought all approaches to diet and / or exercise were created equal, but after almost 20 years as a fitness professional, I've seen people lose fat with everything from kettlebells to kickboxing and others gain muscle employing equally varied approaches.

So what's the secret that separates the winners from the losers? The success stories from the sadly disappointed? …It's mental toughness. The same thing that allows a marathoner to finish the last mile or the football player to finish the fourth quarter when they're both running on fumes, is what allows people like you or me to achieve our fitness goals.

In the broadest sense, mental toughness can be defined as the ability or willingness to maintain the focus and determination to complete a course of action despite difficulty or consequences—to never quit, period. It's something that's valued as much as speed or power in the athletic world. The ability to handle adversity was something that I valued in recruiting during my days as a college baseball coach and a trait that I worked hard to develop in my time as a collegiate and professional athlete. And that same mental toughness or ability to handle adversity is what will be the difference maker for you in the gym – more than the next great training system or diet ever could.

Some will tell you that mental toughness is an innate quality that can't be trained or developed, and while I agree that some people come by it more readily than others – due to the circumstances they've been dealt – that certainly doesn't mean that someone can't become better equipped to focus in on, push through, and overcome the obstacles on their path to success.

So the question is this: How can YOU get mentally tougher? Read on and you'll be better equipped to get more out of whichever program, plan or diet that you choose.

Motivation Is Key – Whenever you find yourself in a tough position and want to throw in the towel, you need to have something you can focus on to provide motivation. For everyone, it's either going to be a success you want to achieve, or a failure you want to avoid. You need to determine which you respond to best.

If you're someone who thinks that you can accomplish anything if you just put your mind to it, then you're motivated to succeed and you simply need to determine exactly what the success you want to achieve is, and hone in on that every time an obstacle pops up in your path. If you're at the other end of the spectrum, the fear of failure is what drives you. Those who fall on this side of the fence seem to respond better to challenges that threaten their self-esteem. It might be a tough thing to accept, but if you fall into this category, the best thing to do when faced with a challenge is to clearly visualize what will happen if you fail and use that as the fuel to get you through.

Either way, **everyone has to find something to focus on for motivation**. If you allow your mind to focus on the pain you may be feeling, or the laziness you want to give in to, you will have a hard time pushing through any adversity.

Show Up – Top achievers show up day after day. The best plan in the world won't help you lose weight or get stronger if you're not putting in the time, day-after–day, to execute it. What happens after you show up is where the real fun begins, but most people can't even make it to that point.

And I'll admit, showing up consistently isn't easy. We all have a million excuses why we can't do something today. …Why we need to wait until Monday to get started. They're all 'crap'. Truth is, if you aren't willing to show up, you don't deserve the results.

So how do you stack the deck in your favor? Workout with someone. It's much harder to stand someone up at the gym than it is to motivate yourself when no one is waiting. Make attendance easy. Find a gym on your route to work or workout at home. Have a routine. We're all creatures of habit, so building your fitness plan into your day will make it much harder to miss a workout.

Get Out Of Your Comfort Zone – Part of building mental toughness involves becoming comfortable performing in stressful situations. One of the best ways you can develop this trait is by consistently doing things you have never done or trying things a different way. We all fear the unknown, and that fear often prevents us from ever developing mental toughness; but by consistently changing up the way that you're challenging your body will help you learn to deal with stress of all kinds.

So if you normally workout at the gym, head outdoors to train for a week. If you typically hop on the treadmill to do your cardiovascular work, try out some bodyweight intervals or find a hill and run some sprints. And don't always feel like you need to color between the lines when it comes to exercise. Arnold Schwarzenagger and his training partners use to carry a barbell out into the woods and take turns doing sets of squats until they were just short of collapse. You don't necessarily need to head to the wilderness to train but taking a sharp deviation from the typical exercises, location or intensity of your workout can break up the monotony, and help take your confidence and motivation to a new level.

Visualize – As a college baseball coach, the first thing our players did when we stepped off the bus to play a game was to find a spot, close their eyes and visualize the success they were about to have in the game. They rehearsed every play, every 'at bat' and every pitch in their minds several times over, imagining exactly how they would feel every step of the way. This dress rehearsal allowed them to feel like they knew what to expect and for their body to simply follow through with the success they'd already enjoyed in their mind.

You should do the same, visualizing every set, every rep, before you ever pick up a weight. If your workout calls for 3 sets of 12 repetitions in the squat with a weight 5 pounds heavier than you've used in the past, you should play the entire process through in your mind, from how you feel as you set up for the first rep to the sensation of pushing through that last rep in the third set. You'll be amazed at how rehearsing the challenges you're about to face beforehand will raise your confidence level and lower your anxiety – as well as help your performance.

Positive Self-Talk – Anytime you step into a challenging situation you're going to have a mental dialogue going on. The environment you're in, the task you're trying to accomplish and your own self-beliefs will blend together and create this mental chatter that is usually split between negative and positive. If you're midway through a challenging workout, there are going to be those voices that creep into your head and tell you that you can't finish, that you aren't strong enough or don't have enough endurance. That you should just give up.

No matter how mentally tough you are, those thoughts or voices will be there. The key is to ignore them and focus on the things that make you believe that you'll be successful. Coach yourself up, remind yourself that 'you can do this' and think about the thing that motivates you that I mentioned earlier. As simple as it sounds, this self talk is often the difference between pushing through and accomplishing your goals and falling just short, because you gave in to the negativity that crept into your mind.

Prepare To Succeed – As a baseball coach I knew that the best strategy on game day was game-like preparation in every practice beforehand. If a player had practiced a situation over and over at game speed, they were much more likely to be successful once the actual competition arrived. This not only meant how they actually practiced an 'at bat' or a pitch, but how they prepared themselves for the greatest chance for success leading to those situations.

In fitness it's the same. Not only should you be preparing yourself for challenging workouts by practicing the proper technique for each exercise, but you should also make sure that you've done the detail work – like making sure you have everything in order ranging from wearing the appropriate shoes for the type of training you're doing, to keeping supportive snacks handy so you don't have to deviate from your nutritional plan.

In the armed forces they say *"The more sweat* used on the *training* field means the *less blood lost* on the battlefield." And while a weight loss plan certainly isn't that way, the importance of preparation remains the same.

Make Adversity Your Ally – In competitive athletics, adversity is what separates the best from the also-rans, and in fitness it's the same. Anyone can excel when things are going smoothly. It's those who respond best once they've hit some bumps in the road that ultimately enjoy the best results.

See, it's never a matter of 'if' there are going to be problems along the way. It's a matter of 'when' they'll arise and how you'll respond. In baseball, the best players quickly move past making an error or a bad call by an umpire, while the rest dwell on those small adversities and let them start a downward spiral. In fitness, the people that reach their goals aren't ones who never miss a workout or slip up on their diet. Instead, they're the ones that don't let one missed workout snowball into a week away from the gym or allow one cheat meal to turn into a dozen.

By knowing that adversity is going to happen and accepting that as part of the journey, you can use it as your ally. Know that one slip up doesn't spell disaster, and that you can jump right back in where you left off, and keep right on toward your goals.

Build A Team – As with most things in life, you will become who you spend time with. So, if you want to get more mentally tough, spend time with people that already are. It's contagious. We continually had players come into our program that performed better as a part of our team than they had in the past, simply because of the culture, the drive and the expectations of the rest of he group. The same type of benefits are just as visible with the recent popularity of fitness bootcamps where people have more accountability, motivation and social support by being part of a group of like-minded and motivated people.

Surrounding yourself with other mentally tough people is a sure way to become mentally tough yourself, so consider finding a motivated work-out partner, joining a good fitness bootcamp (email me at patrigsby@ gmail.com and I'll personally direct you to one) or even join a supportive group online. There's no quicker way to become more mentally tough than having someone there to hold you accountable.

Mental toughness isn't about being a Navy SEAL or even running a marathon. It's about pushing yourself when you want to quit and reaching heights that you didn't think possible. It's about doing another set when your legs are burning, heading to the gym when you'd much rather hit the snooze button, and doing the things others aren't willing to do. So spend some time working to improve your mental toughness, and you'll quickly find that everything else will be improving at the same time.

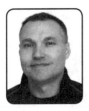

ABOUT PAT

Pat Rigsby is an author, consultant and fitness entrepreneur as well as the Co-Owner of over a dozen businesses within the fitness industry. His company, the Fitness Consulting Group, is the leading business development organization in the fitness industry, the Fitness Consulting Group. This company provides resources, coaching programs and consulting to give you everything you need to start or grow your personal training or fitness related business.

In addition to his business coaching and consulting work, Pat is also the Co-Owner of two of the leading youth fitness and sports performance companies in the world, Athletic Revolution and the International Youth Conditioning Association.

Athletic Revolution, this fastest growing youth fitness and sports performance franchise in the world, was founded due to the need to provide fitness professionals, who sought to serve the Youth Fitness & Sports Performance market, with a systematic approach to developing a successful business that could provide them with the type of career they are seeking, while allowing them to have a profound impact in their community – serving the youth market. You can learn more about the Athletic Revolution Opportunity by going to www.MyAthleticRevolution.com.

The International Youth Conditioning Association is the premier international authority with respect to athletic development and youth-participant-based conditioning. An organization that validates research and provides appropriate examples of practical application for working with young athletes and youth participants at large, the IYCA's goal is to enhance the knowledge of youth sports/fitness professionals and volunteers throughout the world via intensive educational opportunities as well as continuing education requirements. You can learn more about the International Youth Conditioning Association by going to www.IYCA.org.

Pat also hosts a number of conferences, webinars and writes a blog and newsletter that reach over 65,000 fitness professionals on the topics of fitness business development, fitness marketing, and other business topics. He has been seen on NBC, ABC, CBS and in the pages of industry publications like Personal Fitness Professional, Club Industry and Club Business International. You can learn more about Pat's coaching programs and products, or download his collection of free business building gifts by going to: www.FitBusinessInsider.com.

CHAPTER 9

WOMEN, MAKE YOUR BREAKTHROUGH

SPECIFIC STRATEGIES FOR WOMEN TO MAKE A BREAKTHROUGH

BY RACHEL COSGROVE
(AUTHOR OF *THE FEMALE BODY BREAKTHROUGH*)

Are you ready to have a breakthrough and figure out finally how to achieve the body you want? I am going to give you the answers to do that. The title of this book, *Total Body Breakthrough* and the title of my recent book *The Female Body Breakthrough* have the word "Breakthrough" in common and that's because my number one priority is to help women make a breakthrough when it comes to their fitness, nutrition and mindset.

Women have it all wrong when it comes to weight loss. The average woman when she joins a gym looks at how many treadmills there are and the aerobics schedule to see if there are classes that fit in her schedule. When women want to lose weight they torture themselves with repetitive movement for hours on end 'spinning their wheels' or 'running to nowhere' like a hamster in a habitrail! If you take a look at all of the women walking on the treadmills, you'll notice none of them have the body most women want. None of them have made a breakthrough.

The problem is that most personal trainers haven't figured it out yet either. They get a female client who hires them to change their body and they think, "Oh man...another one of those stupid toning programs in the ladies only section with the pink dumbbells doing lots of reps..." Most trainers don't realize that they need to challenge women to get their bodies to change, and to stop being afraid of pushing her to gain muscle to boost her metabolism and to change the way her body looks, permanently.

This chapter will be the answer to what you are looking for – if you are a woman who has been frustrated, struggling to lose weight and get the body you want, and have subjected yourself to any of the following:

- Endless hours of cardio or aerobics classes
- Avoiding strength training because you don't want to get "big and bulky" or maybe you have been told to use some 'rinky dink' pink dumbbells to "tone" for lots of reps
- Cut back your diet to practically starve yourself
- Obsessing about a number on the scale, focusing on a certain weight you want to be and letting the scale make or break your day

WHAT WORKS ABOUT THIS PLAN: NOTHING!
WHAT IS WRONG WITH THIS PLAN: EVERYTHING!

With the above advice, you might lose weight but it will be a mixture of muscle, water and maybe some fat so you'll end up looking like a smaller version of your same self; in the process you will have dropped your metabolism so there will be no way you can keep the weight off and will gain it back guaranteed. This is the cycle most women have been through many times throughout their lifetime. Yet, when they want to lose weight they do the same thing again. The definition of insanity is to do the same thing over and over and expect a different result.

Don't worry if you have been making the mistake of following the above without seeing results and are frustrated and ready to give up. This chapter will give you the answers to FINALLY achieve the lean, toned physique you want – in as little time as possible.

WEIGHT LOSS PROGRAM THAT WORKS!

- Metabolically demanding full body strength training program lifting challenging weights as the priority workout 2-4 days a week.
- Boost your intensity and drop the duration on their cardio sessions performing interval style workouts for no more than 30 minutes at a time.
- Fuel your body with healthy food every couple hours getting your metabolism revving.
- Focus on how your clothes fit and how you look and feel and not on a number on the scale. Focus on Fat Loss, not Weight Loss and completely reinvent your body making a breakthrough.

WHAT WORKS ABOUT THIS PLAN: It will boost your metabolism, it will change your body, it will make you feel confident about yourself, you can eat and you will be able to maintain your new body long term!

WHAT IS WRONG WITH THIS PLAN: NOTHING!

To really change their bodies permanently, women need to start checking out the strength training floor. They need to get out of their comfort zone and push their bodies beyond what it is used to. No more walking to nowhere on the treadmill! I am not talking about bodybuilding routines where you split up each body part and 'bomb and blitz' the pecs or pump up the biceps. It is not necessary for a woman to isolate any muscle group to get the defined look she wants.

Instead, a woman should do a full body, metabolically-demanding program in which she alternates between an upper body compound-movement such as a push up or chin up with a lower body compound-movement such as a squat or lunge. Keep the rest periods short and use a weight that is challenging. Use 3-4 pairs of exercises working out for no more than an hour at a time.

The woman with toned arms and defined legs looks that way because she has the very thing most women are terrified of, muscle. They are so afraid to lift weights in fear of bulking up that they never get their bodies to look the way they want them to. They have it deeply seeded in their subconscious that as soon as they touch anything over 10 pounds, they will sprout humungous muscles! Even if they do use weights, they probably still aren't lifting heavy enough and pushing themselves hard enough to get the look they want. Most women don't know what their bodies are capable of and tend to not push themselves hard enough. There was actually a research study done on this where they showed that women when left to train on their own, lifted loads below what they were capable of.

Maybe it is because women have been conditioned their whole lives to exercise from the point of view of what we "can't" do, rather than what we can do. Women grew up doing "girl" push ups, because we were told we "can't" do actual push ups or hang from the bar instead of a chin up because girls "can't" do chin ups. The first woman to run the marathon had to sneak-in dressed as a man because women "can't" run a marathon, and that was only in the 70's, not that long ago. Women "can't" lift too heavy, they will hurt themselves. We still subconsciously hold ourselves back when it comes to training whether we realize it or not. We need to start training from the standpoint of: What **CAN** you do? How much **CAN** you lift? How strong **CAN** you get? And stop letting "can't" enter our vocabulary. As women start to push themselves in the gym, lifting weights and building lean muscle tissue, their metabolisms will be revving and they will be the toned, defined body they have always wanted.

So how do you get your body to change and make that breakthrough? You have to lift enough weight to build muscle to increase your metabolism, fuel your body with healthy food and turn your body into a fat burning machine. Stop pounding your body with hours of cardio and stop starving yourself! Fuel your body with nutritious foods and follow this program for 8 weeks – and you'll be on your way to a fit and fabulous body you can maintain for life.

The following 8-week program will get you started on your journey to get the body you want. For more programs, information and motivation check out my book, *The Female Body Breakthrough* (published November 2009, Rodale), for a 16-week program to follow when you finish this program. In addition, for continued support go to: www.thefemalebody-breakthrough.com.

THE PLAN

All Exercise Descriptions, pictures and videos can be found at: www. thefemalebodybreakthrough.com/public/totalbodybreakthrough.cfm

This is a two phase program lasting you 8-12 weeks. You can do each phase for 4-6 weeks. Perform the Strength Program twice a week and the Metabolic circuit twice a week. Rest 3 days a week.

WARM UP – Use this warm up before every single workout.

Squat to Stand 10X
Standing Overhead Reach 10X
Alternating High Knee 10X
T-stab Rotation 10X
Side to side step touch 10X
Single Leg Reach 10X

STRENGTH: Strength training is the most important component of a fat loss plan. The routines in this section are designed to boost your metabolism, build lean body mass and burn a ton of calories not only during the workout but for the next 24-48 hours following your workout. It is important that you stick to the reps, sets and rest periods and challenge yourself with loads that you can still maintain your form with, but challenging enough to work your muscles. The more intense your workout, the more you will benefit from the after-burn effect it will create.

PHASE ONE STRENGTH PROGRAM WEEKS ONE TO FOUR

PERFORM TWICE A WEEK FOR 4-6 WEEKS

Perform Warm Up

1A- Clam	1-2 sets	10ea	rest 30s
1B- Prone Cobra	1-2 sets	10(hold 3s each)	rest 60s
2A- Bird Dog	1-2 sets	10ea	rest 30s
2B- Side Plank	1-2 sets	10 (hold 3s each)	rest 60s
3A- Stationary Lunge	1-2 sets	15ea	rest 30s
3B- Bent Over Row	1-2 sets	15	rest 60s
4A- Step Up	1-2 sets	15ea	rest 30s

4B- Incline Push Up	1-2 sets	15	rest 60s
5A- Lateral Lunge	1-2 sets	15ea	rest 30s
5B- L-Lateral Raise	1-2 sets	15	rest 60s

FINISHER – 20 Body weight squats (Rest however long it took you) Repeat 2-5 times. Add a set each week.

PHASE TWO STRENGTH PROGRAM WEEKS FIVE TO EIGHT

PERFORM TWICE A WEEK FOR 4-6 WEEKS AFTER YOU HAVE DONE PHASE ONE FOR 4-6 WEEKS

Perform Warm Up

1A- Prone Hip external Rotation	1-2 sets	10ea	rest 30s
1B- Prone Cobra	1-2 sets	60s hold	rest 60s
2A- Plank with Alt arm reach	1-2 sets	10ea	rest 30s
2B- Side Plank with rotation	1-2 sets	10	rest 60s
3A-Single Leg Romanian Deadlift	2-3 sets	8-10ea	rest 30s
3B- Core stability single arm row	2-3 sets	8-10ea	rest 60s
4A- Lateral Lunge w/ Overhead Press 2-3 sets		8-10ea	rest 30s
4B- Wide Grip Pulldowns		8-10	rest 60s
5A- Dynamic Lunge	2-3 sets	8-10ea	rest 30s
5B- Push Ups Flat	2-3 sets	8-10	rest 60s

Finisher – 20 bodyweight squats, 20 bodyweight squat jumps. Rest as long as it took. Repeat 2-5 times(every week add another set).

METABOLIC INTERVAL CIRCUITS:

This is next on the list of priorities for fat loss. If you only have two hours a week only do the above strength programs and do not do the metabolic circuits. If you have 3-4 hours a week perform this metabolic interval circuit 1-2 times a week. Interval training won't give you the lean body mass benefit that weight training does but it will give you the metabolic boost to increase your metabolism and crank up the calorie burning.

Perform the following 1-2 times a week.

CIRCUIT: This workout uses a jump rope or kettlebell swings as the interval. If you do not have either of these you can do the interval on a cardio machine or as *hill sprints*. The goal = get your heart rate up for the recommended amount of "work" time. Really make sure you are pushing your intensity.

Perform the Warm Up First

THE WORKOUT:

Warm up 3 to 5 minutes using the above warm up

Workout for the "rounds" given below

Week 1-2: 20s high intensity work, 40s Recover, Repeat for 5 rounds, REST 3 minutes and Repeat 5 rounds again.

Week 3-4: 30s high intensity work, 30s Recover, Repeat for 6 rounds, REST 3 minutes and Repeat 6 rounds again.

Week 5-6: 40s high intensity work, 20s Recover, Repeat for 7 rounds, REST 3 minutes and Repeat 7 rounds again.

Week 7-8: 40s high intensity work, 20s Recover, Repeat for 8 rounds, REST 3 minutes and Repeat 8 rounds again.

Week 9-10: 40s high intensity work, 20s Recover, Repeat for 9 rounds, REST 3 minutes and Repeat 9 rounds again.

Week 11-12: 40s high intensity work, 20s Recover, Repeat for 10 rounds, REST 3 minutes and Repeat 10 rounds again.

STEADY STATE CARDIO:

Last priority when it comes to fat loss is using steady state cardio. This type of workout will burn a couple hundred calories while you are doing it but won't create the after-burn effect. Your body also adapts pretty quickly to this type of cardio so we won't put this in until the last two to four weeks. If you have extra time and feel that you are recovering from your strength and metabolic workouts, and want to add in a 5th workout – you can add in one steady state cardio workout of no more than 30-60 minutes of an activity of your choice.

After following the above program for 8-12 weeks you should be making your breakthrough, feeling fit and fabulous and ready to continue your journey. Be sure to pick up a copy of The Female Body Breakthrough for more programs and advice and visit: www.thefemalebodybreakthrough.com.

Websites:
www.thefemalebodybreakthrough.com
www.rachelcosgrove.com
and Co-Owner of Results Fitness: www.results-fitness.com

ABOUT RACHEL

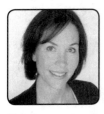

Rachel Cosgrove is the best selling author of The Female Body Breakthrough (published by Rodale November 2009) and is a fitness professional who specializes in getting women of all ages into the best shape of their lives. She owns and operates Results Fitness with her husband in southern California. She has a BS in Exercises Physiology and earned her CSCS from the National Strength and Conditioning Association. She has competed in fitness competitions, is an Ironman triathlete and has set a powerlifting record. She has her own column in Women's Health Magazine and has also been featured in More Magazine, Real Simple, Muscle and Fitness Hers, Shape Magazine, Fitness Magazine, Men's Health, Men's Fitness and Oxygen. She has also had TV appearances on Fox, ABC and WGN. She is on a mission to help as many women make a breakthrough as she can. For more information on Rachel visit: www.rachelcosgrove.com. And for more information on her book and belonging to her community of Fit Females go to: www.thefemalebodybreakthrough.com.

CHAPTER 10

PLAY FITNESS… THE TRUE ESSENCE OF MEGA-FAT BURNING & 'KICK-ASS SHAPE' FOR LIFE

BY BRIAN GRASSO

L et me give you a brief rundown so you know who you're dealing with here.

I'm known as the 'Youth Guy'.

For the past 10 years, I have worked in the trenches with young athletes and youth fitness participants all over the globe. Canada, the United States, Sweden, Italy, New Zealand, Australia; you name it, I've traveled there as the 'know-it-all-guru' for all things kids.

I even started my very own Youth Fitness Organization (the International Youth Conditioning Association) to teach and certify other Fitness Professionals worldwide.

So how does this qualify me to write a chapter about your dilemma – 'How to drop fat and get in the best shape of your life as an adult?' Well, it doesn't really. But read on…

Before I started working exclusively with young people, my job was to improve the sporting performance of some of the greatest athletes in the world. I'm talking Olympians, National Team Competitors, Professional All-Stars and Collegiate Standouts. From Downhill Skiers and Hockey Players to Figure Skaters and Martial Arts Competitors – I trained them all.

And if you think about it, not only do world-class performers all possess incredible athletic skill, they are almost always chiseled from stone. They look great, have low body fat percentages and are in as 'kick-ass-shape' as anyone could ever hope to be.

So, it's the roots of my career that have given me the knowledge to help you in your quest. But beware; I won't be suggesting any form of 'sets and reps', any type of the latest 'fad equipment' and certainly no 'just-take-this-pill' to get you where you want to be, advice.

All I need from you is about 20 minutes, 3 times per week. Yes, that's it and I'm not joking.

But first, a little background is needed…

The primary principles on which Youth Fitness and Elite Athlete Performance are based, is surprisingly similar. They both require related elements of training and these elements are precisely what you need from a 'body fat reduction' standpoint.

The key to understanding your own fitness goals is to understand how the human body works and what stimulus is most effective at producing an adaptation. "Adaptation" is industry lingo that refers to your body going through forced changed as a result of the exercise stimulus you present to it. Important to note here, is that 'hard' does not necessarily equate to 'better'.

It has become a fitness industry caveat to sell consumers on one of two notions:

1. That exercise has to be grueling and cause near-cardiac arrest in order to be worthwhile
2. That exercise can be incredibly easy and limited in both time

and intensity, yet still lead to desired results

Neither are correct. In fact, somewhere right in the middle is the true key.

Let's start with the first myth: **The Too Hard Syndrome**

Should exercise be challenging? Yes. But should it leave you feeling as though you just fought three rounds against Tyson? Absolutely not. Thus, the middle ground.

The fact is that exercise and following a healthy exercise program is as much mental as it is physical. The human organism is built on the reality of Kaizen. This fundamental principle implies that in order to create change, we must enter into the 'newness' slowly, methodically and with a long-term vision in mind. The sage quality of this advice is in remarkable contrast to the standard infomercials and fitness advertisements you commonly see that inundate you with messages like "Lose 30 lbs in 30 days" or "Drop a Dress Size in One Week".

These marketing ploys tend to work because they hit at the nerve of what we all want from a superficial level – Immediate Change... Now! But these programs are seldom effective and when they are, the results are extremely short-lived. That's because they oppose the natural order and law of Kaizen. They require you to delve much too far outside your comfort zone for you to embrace them as part of a new life, or a new way of living.

Additionally, and more to the point, they are entirely 'too hard' for you to maintain the pace required. After a period of time with limited to no exercise whatsoever (which is where most adults find themselves) any type of rigorous training plan will cause adverse adaptations that drop you well beneath what's known as 'normal biological level'. On the surface, you will experience pain, fatigue, decreased range of motion and lethargy. From a physiological perspective, you will go through central nervous system weariness, acute soft tissue trauma and massive alterations in both blood flow and regularity. The point is simple – although the spirit may be strong and want to push again tomorrow, the body and brain will be pleading with you to STOP!! This is a standard issue facing many elite athletes and is known as 'over-training syndrome'. It occurs when the stimulus placed on the body far outweighs the body's ability to compensate properly (or create healthy adaptations).

Now, the converse is true with the second myth: **The Too Easy Syndrome**

Let's be frank here; Eight minutes a day won't cut it. Neither will a cool machine that promises a bikini body in just 9-easy-steps.

But that's not necessarily because the time frame is too inadequate (remember… I promised just 20 minutes, 3 times per week), it's because the intensity or directed load isn't significant enough to cause adaptation.

The extreme science of the matter notwithstanding, the basic philosophy of this issue can be summed up rather easily. The human body was made to move. It is built for movement and requires movement daily to maintain health and functionality. Now, this has nothing to do with 'burning calories' – which has become the lynchpin for most of the modern day prognosticators of fitness. Caloric consumption is NOT what you need to be after here. Systemic (whole body) movement is, and any advice to the contrary should be considered part of the 'Too Easy Syndrome'.

Yes, it is better to park your car at the back of the lot and walk a touch farther to the elevators at work every morning, but that is simply far too easy a stimulus on the body and will absolutely not lead to real adaptations. And before you get defensive because the co-worker in the cubicle beside you 'lost 10 pounds' using the famed Parking Lot Method for weight loss, let me explain this:

1. As a society, we must stop underestimating what the human body is capable of. Measuring your fitness in pounds lost or numbers of calories consumed is not even close to an accurate portrayal of what you can (and should) do in terms of fitness. The human body is an absolute machine of physicality and should be treated as such. Dropping 10 pounds will, and I apologize for the bluntness of this comment, *likely still leave you overweight* and most certainly will leave you in the category of 'not functional' as it relates to human potential from a physical standpoint.
2. The human body must move to be functional – And I don't mean simply 'walk'. Movement is based on joint actions (directions that the joints in your body are able to move) as well as planes of motion (directions we are able to travel). Very simply, the human body is capable of pushing, pulling, changing levels (squatting, bending, lunging) and rotating. A quality exercise program that

is 100% guaranteed to drop the pounds forever AND keep you healthy as you age simply must include all of those features.

So, lets' bring this back around to the whole concept of elite athlete training, the synergies it has when training kids and how that all applies to you…

The two common characteristics that comprise training for both elite and young athletes alike are the two factors that you need to understand with respect to your own fitness goals.

And they are easily summarized in this simple acronym: **M.D.**

M = MOVEMENT MUST DOMINATE

I set up the reveal for this factor above. No matter your goal – fat loss, weight reduction, 6-pack abs or health and functionality – the key to it all is movement in a multi-directional and multi-planar way.

And at the risk of sounding redundant, let me remind you what that means:

Push
Pull
Change Levels
Rotate

All of those movements must be part of a daily (or few times weekly) manifesto of exercise.

Now, in case you hadn't already done the math, this reality implies that exercise equipment, of any kind, is not necessary. You simply don't require it and the best proof of that (in terms of what a human being's body truly wants and needs) is to observe children in their natural environments.

Kids move. Constantly. This desire to play, run, skip, hop, throw things and climb is not a product of 'ants-in-the-pants' or any other form of contemporary 'illness' as defined by modern society (A.D.D., for example). The neurology of human growth and development shows that during the young periods of life, the central nervous system (CNS) is in constant 'gathering' mode.

As young people, we are learning. Our bodies, governed by our CNS, are wired to explore movements, environments and situations. Kids don't mean to 'get into things' – they are being instructed to by an ever-changing, always-learning CNS that is requiring continual input. Not only should this reality be honored and respected, it MUST be enhanced within the training systems of young athletes.

If an adult exercise program involves moving and producing force through an unregulated and free manner, then you are most assuredly on the right track. Run, jump, throw, kick, hop, skip… That kind of stuff.

I know. Doesn't sound like 'normal' fitness advice does it?

But these are the realities of human organisms – movement is the key to fitness and health. And if you doubt me, head outside with a piece of chalk tomorrow. Draw a hop-scotch table on the sidewalk (remember that game?). Inside of 10 minutes, I guarantee you will be breathless, exhausted and more tired than you could possibly imagine…. Give it a try ☺

D = DON'T TRAIN… LEARN

Odd advice, isn't it? I'm asking you to ignore everything you've ever learned (or been sold) about fitness:

- ✓ How many reps leads to 'bulk' versus 'toning'
- ✓ How many calories burned are needed to lose weight
- ✓ How many minutes on a treadmill is necessary for fat loss

Ignore it. Ignore it all.

I don't want you to train or exercise… I want you to learn.

This is a science known as 'motor erudition' and it involves a critical factor called 'physical intelligence'. Contrary to popular belief, the term intelligence doesn't just refer to mental aptitude. It includes the capacity of your body and its ability to move with efficiency and effectiveness.

We can look at this from a mathematical equation standpoint. Walking for an hour will burn somewhere between 175 – 250 calories depending on your speed and body weight. You will also receive the auxiliary benefits (although important) of increasing bone density with minimal impact on your cardiovascular health. But that's it. And trust me, in terms of human capacity, health and real fat loss, that isn't nearly enough.

Now, what if we took the 4-pillars of movement I outlined above and designed a very simple, rotating circuit:

ROUTINE A

Standing Push-Ups against a Tree (10 in a row)
Squatting Pulls using a Fence (10 in a row)
Walking Squats (3 steps, 1 squat for 20 feet)
Squatting Rotations (10 each way)

By performing those exercises back-to-back-to-back-to-back with no rest, pausing for 30 seconds and then repeating the whole circuit for a total of 3 rotations, we would cut our exercise time down to about 10 – 12 minutes and burn in the neighborhood of 2 or 3 times more calories.

Better still, we would be moving in all facets of human motion possible, enhancing ranges of natural motion, improving systemic (whole body) strength and improving elements of coordination such as balance, kinesthetic differentiation and movement adequacy – all of which are important physical elements that when maintained through a lifetime, dramatically reduce the risk of injury and disease.

And that's an example of a very rudimentary, easy circuit. What if you're in much better shape already and just looking for an added push to really give you that 6-pack?

Try something like this:

ROUTINE B

Push-Ups (20)
Sprint to Tree (30 feet)
Pull-Ups on Low Branch (5 – 10)
Squat Jumps (15)
Lunge Walk (30 feet)
Reverse Ab Curls (30)

No rest between exercises; 30 seconds rest between sets; Repeat 5 times.

That will take about 20 minutes and absolutely kick your butt!!

Now, the whole notion of getting from 'Routine A' to 'Routine B' speaks to the factor of "Don't Train… Learn". What we need to progress from one to the other is not necessarily increased fitness or strength, it's increases in body awareness and physical intelligence.

The more you become intelligent with respect to physicality, the more advanced the exercise stimulus is that you can perform and the more your body will adapt to that stimulus.

Things like jumping on one leg, performing 180 or 360 degree rotations while jumping or connecting several highly complex exercises together is directly tied to how physically intelligent you are.

Thus the conclusions that can and will change your life forever are easy:

1. Don't think short-term. Enjoy the process of learning how to move again and then progress to learning more advanced styles of movements – the fitness and body benefits you reap will blow you away
2. Move. In every way you can think of. Don't be content to just lift some weight or walk/run on a treadmill – that is NOT how the human body was meant to gain fitness
3. Get outside for your training. Use your backyard or head to a local park. The environment will be exhilarating and fun and the apparatus you can use (trees, fences, benches, swing-sets) will contribute to your imagination and physical intelligence
4. And remember this one…. Your Mom was right – Just play!!

In case you're wondering, this kind of training is EXACTLY what I used with Olympic and Professional athletes….

Hard to argue with those results!

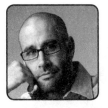

ABOUT BRIAN

Brian Grasso is the Founder and CEO of the International Youth Conditioning Association.

A well-known, respected and outspoken leader in the youth athletic development industry, Brian has written feature articles for sport training magazines throughout North America, including Men's Fitness, Men's Health, Sporting Kid, American Track & Field and Personal Fitness Professional. Brian also contributes to the monthly British sport training publication, Successful Coaching.

An accomplished presenter, Brian provides educational seminars covering youth athletic development and training topics to sporting organizations throughout the world. The list of governing bodies Brian has presented to includes: the National Coaching Education Program, the National Alliance for Youth Sports, the United States Figure Skating Association, the Illinois Olympic Development Program, Skate Canada, the Canadian Athletic Therapists Association and the Korean Aerobic Association among many others. Brian also serves as an educational consultant to the Children's Memorial Hospital's Institute for Sports Medicine.

Brian began his sport-training career as a Performance Coach to Olympic, professional and elite athletes. He has worked with several professional and Olympic athletes from a variety of sports, and has traveled extensively throughout North America and Europe as a Conditioning Consultant for both the Canadian and United States National Team athletes.

CHAPTER 11

'DEATH CAMP'

BY MARC KENT

P eople have always come to me for advice when they want a really hard-core training session. I think it's because I was a Royal Marines Commando for seven years. In the Marines, I learned just how hard the human mind can push the body and I worked out that what we perceive as our limits are mostly psychological. I joined the Marines because I wanted to stretch my own limits and see how hard training could get. In truth, I liked the idea of the whole physical and mental challenge. There were many times in the forces when I thought I couldn't go on, couldn't complete an exercise or just wasn't tough enough. I quickly discovered that, if I thought positive, I'd surprise myself. I had no choice and I learned the hard way. So now, as a certified Master Personal Trainer, I can pass on the lessons I learned in the Marines to clients who do have a choice, and have chosen to train hard and smart to get incredible results. Just like me, my clients find out that if they think they can do it, they can, and they have the life-changing results to prove it.

I was a Royal Marines Commando for seven years and trained hard. I learned a lot about myself and the human body, but I ended up getting injured. As a result, I can no longer run any distance or do any training which places significant impact through my joints. Most people would take those facts and turn them into excuses, using them as reasons for not training hard and only ever getting mediocre results. That's not good enough for me, nor is it good enough for my bootcamp clients. I know that you don't need to do long runs to keep your body fat low, and you don't need to do high impact exercises to build speed and strength. As my most popular circuits and bootcamp sessions prove, anyone can get phenomenal results with body-weight exercises which can be done outside. The most running my circuits clients do with me is 100 metres.

When I left the Marines, I had to develop a system of training which kept me fighting fit without stressing my injuries. Over time, I developed the bootcamp circuits I use with my clients and I now actually feel fitter than I did when I was in the Royal Marines. The ultimate circuit, and the one which my clients have to qualify to do, is the 'Death Camp.' I'll run you through it.

Before we do that, let me tell you a little bit about how 'Death Camp' came to be. Over time, my regular bootcamp clients started wanting more. They were ready for a tougher challenge, something more involved than a regular circuit, a training session I could do with them. "Can't we do something really hardcore?" they asked me. Some of them suggested that I give them a circuit session similar to the training I had done as a Marine. What a challenge that would be! Of course, most Marines training is on an obstacle course, with climbing, sprinting and ropes but I was able to develop a circuit which works on the same principles: upper body, lower body, sprints and body-weight exercises. 'Death Camp' is just 59 minutes long but it works the entire body, building strong, sleek and lean muscles. It blasts body-fat and jacks up the metabolism so that my clients' bodies demand extra calories all day long. It's hard work, but it gets results, and that's why I want to share it with you.

As you can imagine, 'Death Camp' isn't just any regular circuit, and not all of my bootcampers are allowed to do it. It's tough and amazingly effective. 'Death Camp' is packed full of functional, full-body movements, most of which use your own body weight as resistance. You won't build huge amounts of muscle, just strong, lean mass which will continue to blast calories long after you've had a shower. The beauty of this circuit lies in the clever way it shuttles blood from your upper body to lower body (and back again). Not only does this have direct muscle benefits but also means the heart has to work hard to push blood between the legs and shoulders. Of course, you'll be working your core as well. By asking your muscles to work as multiple body parts, you'll ramp up the anabolic effect of exercise, burning as much body fat as you can and massively increasing EPOC (excess post-exercise oxygen consumption). Your entire body will get massive amounts of work done in a short amount of time (although it might not seem short whilst you're doing it!). You'll be hitting all the major muscle groups (and lots of the minor ones) from every possible angle.

'Death Camp' has become a rite of passage for my clients. Before I let them join, they have to be able to perform all the exercises with good form. I pair them up, so they can spot each other and motivate their partners to keep going. Only the best and most hardworking of my clients get to give 'Death Camp' a go. They even get a t-shirt to show they've passed the test! Now here's your chance to join the 'Death Camp' circuit crew (but without the t-shirt, I'm afraid). Are you ready? Grab some water – it's a bit hardcore.

'Death Camp' is 59 minutes long and consists of two circuits of four exercises each before a "finisher" of another four exercises. It's best to do it outside, on a level surface like a flat playing field, empty car park or even your garden if there's enough space. You need at least 50 metres of clear space for the shuttle runs and enough extra room for all the various exercises. Make sure you're well hydrated beforehand, and have plenty of water with you.

WARM UP (5 MINUTES)

First we do a dynamic warm up which should take around five minutes:

10 repetitions of multi-directional lunges (forward, lateral and reverse, each with a difference reach-pattern) followed by a set of 10 press ups, 10 rotating T-planks and 10 mountain-climbers.

We repeat that little lot twice.

We then do some shuttle-run sprints of 50 metres to get the legs firing.

CIRCUIT ONE (16 MINUTES)

Then it's straight into circuit one. For each exercise, work for one minute (as 50 seconds work, 10 seconds rest). Repeat the circuit four times, for a 16 minute section.

1 – deadlifts, using a trap bar (which is easier to use and hits more muscles than a regular free-weights bar). I'll lift 100 kgs for this and be getting 18-20 reps in 50 seconds.

2 – alternating standing dumbell shoulder presses, using as heavy a weight as you can manage. This exercise is all about building muscle endurance: male clients will tend to use 25 kgs whilst female clients average 12.5 kgs.

3 – reverse dumbell lunges

4 – renegade rows

This exercise won't build lots of mass but it will 'torch' major amounts of calories, because we're shunting blood from the lower body to the upper body over and over again.

REST (1 MINUTE)

Take a one minute rest. You're going to need it.

CIRCUIT TWO (16 MINUTES)

Then it's straight into second circuit. For each exercise, work for one minute (as 50 seconds work, 10 seconds rest). Repeat the circuit four times, for a 16 minute section.

1 – chin ups, or another version of a row if you can't manage chin ups with good form

2 – double kettlebell snatches

3 – lateral dumbell deadlifts

4 – elevated press-ups, with your legs on a bench or your hands on dumbbells

Like the first circuit, this section switches between full upper-body exercises, to full body exercises, hitting the glutes, hamstrings, quadriceps and shoulders. It will also work shoulder stability and core strength. The structure of the exercises makes sure you're really firing the upper body, then pushing the blood back into legs – time and time again.

REST (1 MINUTE)

Take a one minute rest. You'll definitely need it by now!

THE FINISHER (12 MINUTES)

We've saved the hardest part till last! Do one minute of each exercise in turn, and repeat the set three times.

1 – 20 single or double kettlebell swings (using a 32kgs or 16kgs bell if you can).

2 – 20 suicide planks: keeping the hips as still as possible, walk up and down from the hands to the elbows.

3 – sprint runs: 50 metres out, 50 metres back.

4 – 20 squat thrusts or mountain-climbers.

This final section ends the circuit with high-intensity cardio to shoot the heart-rate through the roof, build speed and agility and inject extra power into the legs, back and core. We do this section for 12 solid minutes with no rest trying to complete as many rounds as possible.

COOL DOWN (8 MINUTES)

Cool down slowly and stretch out by walking in a large circle, performing upper-body stretches as you walk: rear shoulders, triceps and the chest. Then stand and stretch the quadriceps, hip flexors and hamstrings, before lying down to stretch the back and hips.

Congratulations! You've just finished 'Death Camp' – the toughest circuit you'll find outside of the Royal Marines.

Go ahead and do the 'Death Camp' on your own or with training partners if you're confident in your ability to complete all the lifts and moves with good form. If you're not, ask a professional to show you how to do them. You can also consider substituting equipment or similar movements, just make sure you are working the same body parts in the same order.

MARC'S TOP TIPS FOR SURVIVING DEATH CAMP:

1. Make sure you're fully warmed up: use the 'Death Camp' warm

up I outlined above, as it's proven to work.

2. Work on your flexibility: as well as stretching, do prehab work using a foam roller.

3. During the main workouts, stay focused and keep pushing. Don't let self-doubt hold you back.

4. It's going to be hard work! What gets me through is counting reps in my head to keep focused. This gives you a goal to match (or beat) next time.

5. Have a positive mental attitude: believe in yourself and believe you can get it done.

6. Hydration is crucial: make sure you're well hydrated before you start the circuit.

7. Eat healthily throughout the day: don't train on an empty stomach or eat too soon beforehand.

8. Afterwards, get high-quality protein and carbohydrates in to help the important recovery phase.

9. Don't forget to stretch and drink lots of water after you've cooled down.

10. Don't do a circuit like this every day, or even every week. I'd recommend doing it once a month, and keeping a record of your reps and weights so you can see yourself improving.

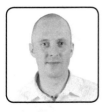

ABOUT MARC

Marc Kent is a qualified Sports Therapist and advanced Personal Trainer with a Masters in Personal Training. He runs a training facility in North Devon, UK, where he coaches clients on a one-to-one, group training and bootcamp basis. Originally from Carlisle, Marc moved to North Devon whilst serving as a Royal Marines Commando.

Marc has trained athletically and played sports since he was a child. At school, he started his own football team and played hockey. However, he always wanted to race motorbikes competitively and did this for two years. He then decided that his fitness goals needed a tougher target and joined the Marines in 2001. His goal was to enjoy the challenge of pushing his fitness to the limit and seeing how much his body could adapt to. Whilst serving as a Royal Marines Commando, Marc sustained an injury, which eventually resulted in him no longer being able to take part in long endurance runs or high-impact exercise.

Despite this limitation, Marc was determined to find a way to remain as fit as he'd been in the Marines. After 7 years in the forces, he left and decided to train to become a PT. He'd always been the person his friends and family turned to for fitness, training and nutrition advice, and wanted to be qualified to give the best advice possible.

Marc had to develop a way to keep very fit without leaning on long cardio sessions. He began to put together his signature programmes incorporating kettlebells, sprint work, body weight exercises and high intensity training.

Marc qualified as a Personal Trainer in 2007 and went on to complete a Masters in Personal Training. Further to that, he studied Sports Therapy, gaining a distinction. He opened his North Devon studio in 2009, offering bootcamps, one-on-one and group personal training, sports therapy, rehabilitation and massage.

Clients all want fat-loss, which Marc's system delivers, but Marc sees a lot of postural problems brought about by sedentary working. All of his programmes are developed to improve posture by using free weights and body weight exercises in a functional way. His bootcamp clients lose, on average, 35lbs over the course and one client lost 56lbs in 6 months!

Marc's philosophy to training is "train hard, eat smart", meaning train as hard as you can and eat foods as close to their natural state 90% of the time. *He feels people should live for now, but keep fit for the future.* His ultimate goal is to be a fitness consultant and mentor for other personal trainers.

CHAPTER 12

FROM FAT KID TO FIT PRO

BY STEVE KREBS

www.thestevekrebsshow.com
315-790-5851
stevenrkrebs@hotmail.com

My name is Steve Krebs, and at one point in my life I weighed over 285 lbs. At barely 6 feet tall (on my tip toes), I wasn't exactly the poster boy for physical fitness. Growing up, I was always the "husky" or "chubby" kid. I played sports, and was always a decent athlete, but unfortunately for me there were always baked goods and treats in the house. There were points in my life when I actually hid food in my room. I had a love affair with food (I still do, but have learned to control it). I was an emotional eater, and I overate at almost every meal. Needless to say, my lack of self control, and unhealthy eating habits caused me to balloon up to 100 pounds overweight. Being overweight made me self conscious, unhappy, and not so popular with the ladies. So, something had to give... because I like the ladies! My battle with overeating and weight continued well into my college years, where I developed a new recipe for body fat: Beer + Late Night Eating + Lack of Exercise + More Beer = Still FAT!!

I truly believe that every unfit person has a breaking point. A moment where being out of shape, unhealthy, and lacking confidence becomes too much to bear. There is a point where you don't want to be called "fat", "chubby", or the plethora of other insults that one becomes accustomed to growing up as a "fat kid". My breaking point occurred when my high school sweetheart kicked me to the curb! I was overweight, depressed, anxious, and just plain old unhappy. All at once I decided to take control of my life. I started eating healthy, and began a vigorous exercise program. I stayed dedicated to my program, and became obsessed with goal setting (the secret to success). I lost over 100 pounds on my own! After studying and becoming obsessed with health and fitness, I changed my college major to Health Science. This change started me on a journey to become the best trainer and fitness professional I could be!

Along my journey, I have compiled seven steps that will help anyone transform their mind, body, and soul. The first seven will get you started on your journey with some actionable tips to improve your life. These seven steps will help you achieve the life and body of your dreams, but the one main ingredient to obtaining goals and looking great is to take action! Everyone has great intentions, but if you do not take action, those intentions will remain exactly that.

7 STEPS TO GO FROM FAT KID TO FIT ADULT!

STEP 1) FIND YOUR MOTIVATION!

Each person has a different motivation to make a life/ behavior change. It cannot be for anyone else but you. Once you find the reason behind your decision to make this change, you MUST remind yourself every morning and every night why you are going to stick with this lifestyle/ behavior change. This ideal must be reinforced over and over again!

STEP 2) RID YOUR LIFE OF NEGATIVITY!

We all have negative things, experiences or people in our lives. If you want to make a change you MUST remove these things from your life. In your journey to change your life you will most definitely find that you have saboteurs that want to stand in your way. Saboteurs are people that for their own selfish reasons, don't want to see you change in a positive way. Remember, *misery loves company*.

STEP 3) SET S.M.A.R.T. GOALS: SPECIFIC. MEASUREABLE.

ATTAINABLE. REALISTIC. TIME ORIENTED.

Make sure to set your s.m.a.r.t. goals for short term and long term goals. The more specific your goals, the more likely you are going to obtain them. Write out all of your goals by hand and post them all over your house, and even tell friends and family members so you will be held more accountable.

STEP 4) TAKE ACTION!

Each day you MUST do something that brings you closer to your s.m.a.r.t. goals. Baby steps are the way to go.

STEP 5) HIRE A PROFESSIONAL.

When starting your fitness program it is very important to enlist the help of a proven fitness professional. Notice I did not say personal trainer! You do NOT want to hire a "weekend warrior" or old school trainer who has ZERO education, and poor credentials. When looking for a good coach, make sure they are college educated in a fitness related field and have some sort of money back guarantee. Also make sure to ask for at least 3 references or testimonials from past clients.

STEP 6) OUT WITH THE OLD AND IN WITH THE NEW!

Bad habits are hard to break, but not impossible. Most experts say it takes 30 days to develop a good habit, but 3 times as long to break a bad one. So let's replace those old habits (eating late, overeating, low self-esteem, low confidence, etc.) with some positive new ones like eating 5-6 small balanced meals a day, exercise at least 5 days a week, and being happy every day! You hold your life in your own hands, choose to be happy and healthy!

STEP 7) REWARD YOURSELF!

The best way to stay dedicated to your new life, body and mindset is to reward yourself along the way. Life is all about the small victories! Every time you obtain one of your s.m.a.r.t. goals you should have a positive reward. The key to the reward is that it needs to go along with your goals. So if weight loss is your goal, your reward shouldn't be an unhealthy behavior (pigging out, smoking, drinking, etc.).

By following these steps you are on your way to an amazing transformation! To help you achieve your fitness goals, I am going to reveal my top 3 workouts that will allow you to burn body fat around the clock. When starting a fitness program there are a few steps you must take:

TOP 3 FAT INCINERATING WORKOUTS

1) "TERRIBLE TABATA'S"

20 seconds of work – 10 seconds of rest
4 Rounds
2 x through each round

This intense circuit requires you to do 20 seconds of work followed by 10 seconds of rest for 4 rounds. Each round consists of completing exercises a-d 2 times. You will get 60 seconds of rest in between each round.

a) KB Swing
b) Mountain Climber
c) KB High Pull
d) Burpee

Exercise Descriptions:

a) Place one kettlebell between your feet. Push back with your butt and bend your knees to get into the starting position. Make sure that your back is flat and look straight ahead. Drive though with your hips explosively taking the kettlebell straight out.

b) Place yourself in the basic push-up position with your arms in line with your chest and your legs extended outward. Rest on the balls of your feet while bringing one leg forward to your chest and back to its original position. Keep the right leg tucked during the forward and back movement of the left leg.

c) Begin in a shoulder width stance. Place kettlebell between your feet. Grip kettlebell with both hands and snap behind your hips. Drive through hips explosively. Pull with elbows above hands.

d) Begin in a standing position. Drop into a squat position with your hands on the floor in front of you. Kick your feet back, while simultaneously lowering yourself into a pushup. Immediately return your feet to the squat position, while simultaneously pushing up with your arms. Leap up as high as possible from the squat position with your arms overhead

2) DENSITY SETS

2 minutes of work
60 seconds of rest
7 rounds
5 reps each exercise

In Density sets, each exercise is done for 5 repetitions in a 2 minute timed set. You will cycle through these four exercises as many times as possible within the 2 minute time limit of each set. This workout consists of 7 rounds. Each 2 minute round is followed by a 60 second rest.

a) One Arm KB Swing- 5 each
b) Running Push Up
c) TRX Row
d) TRX Suspended Crunch

Exercise Descriptions:

a) Place one kettlebell between your feet. Push back with your butt and bend your knees to get into the starting position. Make sure that your back is flat and look straight ahead. Drive though with your hips explosively taking the kettlebell straight out.

b) Begin in a push up position. Perform 1 Push Up, then alternate driving each leg into a mountain climber.

c) Use Neutral Grip on the TRX. Squeeze shoulder blades together as you row your bodyweight forward.

d) Place feet in bottom stirrups of TRX. Hands Shoulder width apart. Raise hips so that they are in line with shoulders. Bring hips towards the ceiling while bringing your knees in.

3) "KILLER CONDITIONING"

30 seconds of work / 30 seconds of rest
5 Exercise Circuit

4 Rounds

"Killer Conditioning" is a 5 exercise circuit consisting of 4 rounds of 30 seconds of work 30 seconds of rest. You will complete 4 rounds of an exercise before moving on to the next. For example, all 4 rounds of the H2H Swing must be completed before moving to the TRX squat jump.

    a) H2H KB Swing
    b) TRX Squat Jump
    c) Burpee
    d) Battling Ropes
    e) V-sit

Exercise Descriptions:

a) **H2H KB Swing** – Place one kettlebell between your feet. Push back with your butt and bend your knees to get into the starting position. Make sure that your back is flat and look straight ahead. Drive through with your hips explosively, taking the kettlebell straight out. At highest point switch hands.

b) **TRX Squat Jump** – Grip TRX with neutral Grip. Feet shoulder width apart. Sit into a squat, then jump explosively. Make sure to land softly into the next repetition.

c) **Burpee** – Begin in a standing position. Drop into a squat position with your hands on the floor in front of you. Kick your feet back, while simultaneously lowering yourself into a pushup. Immediately return your feet to the squat position, while simultaneously pushing up with your arms. Leap up as high as possible from the squat position with your arms overhead.

d) **Battling Ropes** – Stand Up as you create large waves with the ropes, once the ropes are overhead drive them back down into the ground as fast as possible.

e) **V-sit** – Begin in a seated position, contract your abdominal muscles and core, and pull your knees into your body. Reach your arms straight forward.

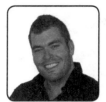

ABOUT STEVE

Steve Krebs is definitely not your typical fitness professional. At one point in his life he weighed almost 300 pounds, and was considered the "fat kid".

In his 10 plus years as a fitness professional, Steve has helped countless people reach their fitness goals and full potential. Steve has been recognized as one of the top fitness professionals and boot camp experts in the world, and anyone that knows him will definitely tell you that he is humble, very calm and level headed......

Steve Krebs is owner and head coach at Next Level Athletic Performance home of Steve Krebs Fitness Boot Camps. (It was ranked 'Top 10' in America... not too shabby huh?). Next Level is located at 9562 River Rd., Marcy, NY 13403 (that is where you will send your fan mail). Steve can be reached at 315-790-5851 or via email at stevenrkrebs@hotmail.com.

Steve's mission in life is to spread health and fitness across the universe while having fun in the process!

Steve Krebs is also creator and "star" of the critically acclaimed "The Steve Krebs Show". The Steve Krebs Show is a web television show that has been compared to shows like "Talk Soup" and "Laguna Beach". As you can see, Steve Krebs is a completely serious human being, with zero sense of humor. He also once wrestled a Grizzly Bear on International Television to a disappointing draw.

Bootcamp info: www.nextlevelbeachbodybootcamp.com

CHAPTER 13

KETTLEBELL TRAINING FOR THE FITNESS PROFESSIONAL

BY PAMELA MacELREE

Kettlebell training has become an increasingly large area of focus in the fitness industry. We have all seen it happen – the novelty of the latest fitness craze not only entices our clients to challenge their bodies in new ways, but temporarily encourages them to get moving more frequently. We have also seen the rise and fall of these trends as the next "hot item" comes along. Kettlebell training is a little different. The kettlebell itself as well as the resulting physical benefits of such training have been in existence since the sixteenth century. The overall shape of the kettlebell as we know it today, more or less a cannonball with a handle, began to take shape near the end of Czarist era in Russia. One of the kettlebell's original uses was as a tool for weights and measures on farms.

I was first introduced to kettlebell training in a local gym a little over six years ago. During my first set of kettlebell swings, I didn't think much beyond the fact that my workout ended up being a lot of fun and I had felt muscle groups I had never used. As I began to recognize the unique physical benefits that the kettlebell can provide, I found myself buying my own kettlebell, then later attending kettlebell workshops, and seeking out the knowledge of those who professed to be kettlebell training experts. At that time I began bringing my own equipment into the gym, trying my best to disregard the strange looks I tended to receive. By then, I was hooked – I needed to know everything I could learn about kettlebell training.

When I discovered kettlebell training, I was working a corporate job that consumed a significant amount of time and I needed workouts that could be done quickly and produced results. I quickly discovered that these workouts could enable me to become strong and lean at the same time, without having to spend endless hours in the gym. The reason for this discovery is that the majority of kettlebell exercises are full body exercises, so there is no isolation work, one of the most time-consuming parts of a standard workout. As a result, you are able to combine simple bodyweight exercises with kettlebell exercises for a head-to-toe workout in half the time of a traditional gym workout.

During the beginning stages of my kettlebell training, I was encouraged by the way my body responded so quickly to the exercises. At the same time, what I started to notice was that many people I saw at the gym didn't appear to be progressing in their physical fitness, and the likely reason was that their workouts never changed. Some people had been trying their workout routine for just a few weeks, and others for almost a year! I couldn't believe it, not noticing a physical change in a year, I would have felt so defeated, not to mention like I had wasted my time.

Prior to working out with kettlebells, I had become accustomed to running for hours on end, day-after-day. I started to get bored with my workouts and started to plateau, and was no longer seeing the results of my training that I had experienced in the beginning. Overall, I needed a change. So I made one – I switched to kettlebell training and weight lifting. I developed a passion for the style of training that changed my body into the strong and lean form I had always aspired to create. It was relatively easy for me to teach myself the exercises and educate myself on a style of training that produced the results I was looking for, such as decreased body fat and an increase in strength and lean muscle mass.

My favorite kettlebell exercises tend to be ones that combine strength training with stability. A great example of this is the windmill and its multiple variations – this movement alone involves upper body and core strength, shoulder stability, and flexibility.

There are several variations of the windmill, creating a variety of programming options. The movement pattern for all of the variations remains the same, however the loading pattern is altered. Three of the more popular windmill variations are: the low windmill where the kettlebell stays in the low hand, the high windmill where the kettlebell resides overhead and demands significant shoulder stability, and lastly the double windmill where one kettlebell is in the low hand and overhead.

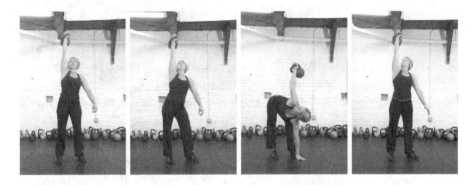

After several months of educating myself on kettlebells, I began to show friends and family the exercises, watching as they benefited in the same ways that I did. On a leap of faith I decided to look into a kettlebell certification course as well as other personal training certifications. I had been an athlete in high school and spent many afternoons in a weight room without a lot of direction; now I was seeing the same thing with adults at the gym. I knew I could do better for them, I knew I was going to try.

I began completing various certifications and working with my clients, helping them to perfect their technique and getting them results, I saw value in helping other people do the same for their clients.

Currently, I work regularly with trainers and coaches to educate them on the cues and techniques that are essential to effective and safe kettlebell training. Some of the biggest mistakes in kettlebell training result from a lack of knowledge of the kettlebell's unique properties along with the implementation of the kettlebell within training programs.

The top three mistakes you can make in implementing kettlebell training into your client's programs are:

1. **Not being able to recognize faulty movement patterns**. Good coaches don't necessarily have to be able to do the exercises they want their clients and athletes to do, but they need to be able to coach them properly. Just like any new training technique, kettlebell training requires instruction, practice and repetition. If you just picked up a DVD and started doing swings last week, then you shouldn't be teaching it to your clients yet. Not being able to diagnose improper movement patterns could result in injury for yourself and your clients. Work one-on-one with a coach who understands proper technique and form.

2. **Avoid over-prescription of repetition and exercises.** It's important to remember that when first implementing kettlebell training, it's new to your clients and athletes, so you want to introduce the kettlebell exercises and volume over time. Teaching your clients and athletes new exercises is beneficial to both their progress and to avoid boredom, and you'll want to add in the appropriate amount of skill work prior to adding the new kettlebell exercises into the workout program. You don't want to show your clients and athletes how to do a new kettlebell exercise one day and then prescribe 200 reps in the next workout.

3. **Mix it up to keep things fresh.** Kettlebell training is an awesome tool to integrate into most training programs, but it isn't the only tool you have in your toolbox. Don't become obsessive and over-program kettlebell training; make sure it fits into the end goals of your clients and athletes.

With proper teaching techniques and cuing you can create valuable and effective kettlebell training programs that produce the health and fitness results your clients are searching for, in significantly less time at the gym than they are used to.

The following kettlebell and bodyweight workout is a great example of a short, full body workout.

1A) Kettlebell Windmills (any variation) 5 x 3/3
2A) Kettlebell Clean and Push Press 4 x 30/30seconds
2B) Kettlebell Romanian Deadlift 4 x 30 seconds
2C) Push Ups 4 x 30 seconds
2D) Kettlebell High Pulls 4 x 30 seconds

2E) Reverse Lunges 4 x 30 seconds

2F) Rest 4 x 60 seconds

It's important to be able to alter workouts based on your client's skill set and ability. In the above workout you would program low windmills in for a beginner client or someone who has minimal to poor shoulder stability. The high windmill and double windmill would be more advanced variations to be prescribed for clients who are more advanced and have good shoulder stability.

In the second part of the workout, it may be more appropriate to have deconditioned clients perform kettlebell presses, good morning stretches, modified push ups (if necessary), high pulls, and reverse lunges. One other option to consider is to decrease the number of sets and/or the length of time that each exercise is completed.

A more advanced client could see more of a challenge by doing clean and jerks, single arm Romanian deadlifts, an advanced push up variation, single arm high pulls, and jumping lunges.

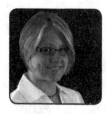

ABOUT PAMELA

Pamela MacElree holds a Bachelor of Science degree from The Pennsylvania State University and is currently completing a Masters of Science in Exercise Science, with a focus on Injury Prevention and Performance Enhancement from California University of Pennsylvania. Pamela is owner of Urban Athlete, which operates a strength and conditioning studio and Brazilian Jiu-Jitsu academy in Philadelphia, Pennsylvania.

Pamela is an independent contractor for one of North America's largest pharmaceutical companies, supplying health and wellness education to its employees. Along with Kettlebell Athletics, she has collaborated on developing and delivering the only peer-reviewed and most comprehensive Kettlebell training certification for Fitness Professionals in the United States and Germany, Pamela has also created training programs for local men and women's rugby and squash teams.

Pamela lives in Philadelphia, Pennsylvania and enjoys workouts in the park with her two rescue dogs, Bella and Leo.

http://PMacStrong.com

CHAPTER 14

THE DIFFERENCE BETWEEN SUCCESS AND FAILURE

BY JOHN O'CONNELL

I first met Vivienne back in January 2010. She had been chosen, as one of 3 (mothers), to appear on a television programme that would document their progress over an 8 week weight loss programme. Vivienne was a diet expert, she told me as we rummaged through her cupboards and refrigerator filming the first episode. She had been on every diet known to man. Soup diets, low fat, low carb... and knew exactly how many points there were in every food item she bought. Some 'worked,' she said. But when I questioned what she meant by 'worked,' I found out she had lost some weight and then put it all back on, with interest. This is the torment of the serial dieter. Lose some weight and gain some more back.

Well, if you gain it all back, then it didn't work!

For Vivienne, weighing in at 226lbs/16 stone 2lbs, those diets definitely didn't work. In fact they made her situation worse.

Anyway, the day ended with me putting all of the healthy food in her house on her kitchen table, in one neat little pile. Seriously, it was tiny! I asked her how she expected to lose weight with so little choice of healthy food and so much junk and highly processed food in the house. Her reply was more startling than the lack of healthy groceries in her kitchen.

"I don't know, but I'll have to try".

"Vivienne" I said in utter shock, "in order to succeed you must give yourself as much choice as possible, surround yourself with as much wholesome food as you can find and get rid of the garbage. You must be prepared to succeed".

I left her with a shopping list and meal plans so she could start to become more prepared each day to finally lose weight and keep it off.

I want to add in right now that during the programme, Vivienne lost 27 lbs in 8 weeks, and is now less than 176 lbs at the time of writing. Most probably around the 170 mark, as I haven't re-assessed her in a few weeks, and every time I do she amazes me with her results!

So, what was different this time that actually worked for her? The programme I had her on was no miracle programme. In fact the programmes in this book are very similar and probably more effective than what I designed for Vivienne. However, that's all very good on paper, but what makes someone succeed while others falter within days of starting?

Well, in order to answer that question I want to share a phone conversation I had with her two days after we initially met.

The first question I asked was, "What do you want?" A seemingly simple question usually followed by an all too simple answer.

"I want to lose weight and tone up".

I've heard this answer way too often and it irritates me to no end! It annoys me because it rolls off the tongue too easily, as if it's going to happen tomorrow.

So I asked her what she meant.

"Well I hate the way I look, and don't want to be this way anymore".

"I asked what you WANT, not what you don't want! In an ideal world, what would you want to look like? How would you feel if you were at a weight you were really comfortable with, and could wear clothes with freedom?"

After a long pause, which there usually is because most people never really think about exactly what they want their lives to be like. They seem to just concentrate on what they don't want or don't like about themselves. She finally answered: "Well, I'd love to be able to fit into my wedding dress again and be the same weight I was then."

She continued to describe how that would make her feel and what she would be able to do being fit and healthy, having all that extra energy to do more things with her kids and husband.

"So, it's much more than just losing weight and toning up?" I asked. I could almost hear the light bulb switching on above her head.

"Yes" she exclaimed with an enthusiasm and excitement in her voice that wasn't there before. "I never really thought about it like that before," she added.

I explained to her that that was one of the reasons why it hadn't worked before. She never really had much motivation to just lose weight and tone up. But thinking about all the amazing changes in her life that could and would happen when she made it, was really exciting.

This was something she actually wanted now. I could even sense it on the phone.

I knew I had her attention so I continued to probe a bit more. It's all very well and good to get excited about something, but that can soon fade away unless there's something else pushing you, something stronger and more emotional.

I asked her what the most important thing in her life was.

Her kids was the easy response.

I then asked who the most important person in her life was.

Her exact words were: "well, I can't choose just one of my 3 kids, so my husband".

"Really?" I asked sarcastically.

"If anything happened to you what would happen to your husband and the kids?"

"Oh, is it me?" She inquired.

"Well, if something happened to you and you couldn't take care of them or look after them how would that make you feel? What would they do?" After this the phone went silent for a moment and when she responded I could hear the emotion in her voice as she tried to hold her tears back.

"John, I don't want to think about that," her voice trembled with sadness.

"But, if you keep going the way you are, something is going to happen and you won't be able to give your children the life they deserve or even be around for them in a few years." It may sound harsh, but she needed to hear this from someone.

"John, you have me crying now" she wept.

As a mother, her maternal instincts were kicking in now and the thought of not being able to provide a great life for her kids was not an option. Becoming fit, healthy and strong was a much better option. Not only to ensure she remained well enough to look after her family but to be able to do more things with them. We discussed this more at length. We talked about what would happen if she didn't change and remained unfit and overweight, or worse, got fatter over the next few years. A scary process but it really makes you re-evaluate your current situation.

There were a lot more tears, but by the end she was a changed woman. She now had the focus needed to ensure that success was the only option. That being there for her family was far more important than eating a bar of chocolate or a pizza.

During Vivienne's transformation she regularly reported the new activities she was discovering she could do – go swimming with the kids, play for hours with them without getting tired and then being able to do the housework afterwards. She could go out for walks to the park and still come home and have time for exercise. Just having more energy and not being wiped out at the end of the day.

These are the little everyday things that actually make a huge difference in the quality of our lives and with our family and friends. They are taken for granted all too often when in fact that's what living is, being able to share quality experiences with the ones we love.

The fact is no one wants to just lose weight and tone up. What we want is to improve the quality of our lives or simply be happier. And figuring out exactly what you want is the most vital step in your success.

Now most people have dreams and wishes of what they want. Some even write them down and call them goals. However goals are not what we think they are! We tend to perceive the outcome we want as a goal. 'I want to lose 50 lbs' ...is not a goal. It's an outcome or a reward, a reward for doing certain things. For example, in order to lose 50 lbs, you must train at least 3 days a week. You will have to change certain eating habits and follow a specific eating plan daily. These behaviours, the things we need to do in order to succeed, are in fact the real goals.

When you think about it, the reward for achieving your goals, going to the gym, eating better, etc., is the loss of 50 lbs, the improved health, being able to shop for clothes with freedom, and looking in a mirror and being happy with what you see.

A goal is in fact a behaviour, not a thing.

If you want to own a Ferrari, you know you will have to work hard and create an income substantial enough to be able to afford one. Once you do this you then reward yourself with the car, the house, etc.

I think most people understand these rules regarding wealth but when it comes to health and fitness they are often ignored. I don't know anybody who dreams of driving a fancy car but doesn't accept the fact that they will either have to work 'damn hard' for it or else it will remain just a dream. And yes, winning the lotto counts as a dream!

When it comes to losing weight, certainly with some of the clients I have consulted with, a lot of people seem to think that it should just magically happen without any effort or sacrifice. They want all the rewards without changing their behaviours. They tell me they don't want to train hard, or they won't give up a certain food, they won't deprive themselves etc. Unfortunately, it doesn't work this way. There must be some work involved to get the rewards.

If it was easy, we'd all be super fit and healthy, …and I'd be out of work!

People rarely set goals, they set their rewards and never actually set or complete the individual goals needed to gain the reward. So, in order to finally succeed, changing your behaviour and setting well-formed goals is without doubt the simplest yet most effective way. Setting daily and weekly goals/tasks/behaviours (whatever you want to call them) is the fastest route to achieving the great rewards that being fit and healthy will bring you.

For example:

Plan out each day what you are going to eat and when. Plan your training sessions over the week, what days, what times and where, and let nothing prevent them from going ahead. Know what you are doing in the sessions (choose a programme from this book and stick with it until it's completed, then move on to the next one).

I now want to show you some practical steps you can use to make your journey really successful. The first thing I do with my clients is ask them what they want, and I keep asking until I really find out what makes them tick. So, some great questions you can start to ask yourself are:

1. What exactly do you want? (In an ideal world and if there were no limitations)
2. When do you want it?
3. What will you look like? (Be really descriptive)
4. How will you feel when you have already achieved this?
5. What will your family, friends and/or colleagues say to you/ about you? (Only positives here, we don't do negatives)
6. What will you be able to do more of?

Now, this isn't just as simple as reading this and thinking some sort of magic is going to happen. These questions, and more importantly, the answers to them, can become a part of your daily routine. Whether you choose to think about them before bed, first thing in the morning or whenever you need more motivation, they will help you stay focused on completing your daily goals. Essentially, you are giving your brain a map to follow. And your destination is the answers to these questions.

The route you take (your goals) on this brain map can be calculated as follows (this is just a rough guideline for you so you can go into more detail):

- How many training sessions are required per week in your programme?
- On what days are you doing these sessions, and at what times?
- What are you going to be eating?
- What foods do you need to avoid?
- How many meals are you eating per day and what are they?
- What time is each meal?

And so on...

These are your real goals! Every time you achieve one of these goals you take a step closer to the rewards you really desire. Every time you skip one you will have taken a step back. The great thing about this is that it's really easy to assess your progress each week. You can simply look back at how many goals you've ticked off and improve it for the next. You can also identify what areas are lacking and improve on them.

I want to leave you with a final thought. Bill Gates, Lance Armstrong, Oprah Winfrey and every other successful person in the world has only succeeded due to the team they surround themselves with.

Lance Armstrong had a team built around him, without which he wouldn't have won the Tour de France 7 times. Oprah can't earn the millions she does without an entire production company helping her, and Bill Gates could never have earned his billions without thousands of employees contributing to Microsoft's success.

So who's on your team? Who can you ask for help and support? Build a great team around you and your journey will be so much easier.

ABOUT JOHN

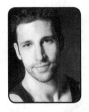

John O'Connell is one of Ireland's leading health and fitness experts. Having extensive experience working as a personal trainer in a wide variety of gyms in Ireland and abroad, John has trained thousands of clients and has also developed many advanced training programmes for fitness staff.

John is regularly featured on Irish Television as a resident health & fitness expert. He is also sought after for radio, newspaper and magazine features. John has worked as a health and fitness consultant for Lyons Tea and SPAR, the world's largest retail chain.

John has an impressive client list. His clients list boasts a number of celebrities and professional organizations, including the Irish Police Force and the New Zealand All Blacks Rugby Team.

As well as working with the NZRFU he has also been involved with many other professional sporting teams including the Ireland A Senior Rugby Team, the European Cup winning Leinster Senior Rugby Team, the Dublin Football Team, Queensland Reds Rugby Team, Murphy and Gunn/Newlyn (a Continental Irish Cycling Team) and the Australian Cycling Team, FRF Couriers.

Along with his numerous exercise and health qualifications John is a licensed Neuro-Linguistic Programming (NLP) Master Practitioner and Life Coach. He is a level 2 internationally certified Strength and Conditioning Coach through PICP and is one of Ireland's few Bio Signature Modulation practitioners.

John walks his talk. He remains in peak physical condition throughout the year and is a former cyclist. He also auditioned with 10,000 others for a contender's role on the UK TV series Gladiators. He was chosen in the top 16 to compete on the show and only a neck injury prevented him from taking it further.

John's ability to motivate and inspire others is outstanding. He has helped transform the lives of others not just through training but through his unique style of mental training using his NLP coaching skills.

By combining physical, mental and nutritional training, John can offer a truly unique service to his clients, one that is matched by none. He constantly strives to learn more by attending seminars and internships with world experts so he can help more people achieve the fitness, health and body that they desire.

To contact him call +353 (0)1 2542120 or email john@newenergy.ie

CHAPTER 15

YOUR MIND/BODY EXPERIENCE

BY GREG JUSTICE, MA

I f you think you can, you're right. If you think you can't, you're right. Henry Ford was right on the money. While you can't control everything that happens to you, you do have 100% control over how you choose to respond and react.

The phrase mind/body has been used most often regarding traditional Eastern exercise methods, such as Yoga, Tai Chi, and Qi Gon. These exercise methods incorporate deliberate body movement with meditative and conscious breathwork components. They highlight alignment, energy flow, inner awareness, balance, flexibility, and more.

Researchers have discovered many amazing things about mind/body health and healing. While there is still much to learn about this subject, your mind and body have a relationship with each other that is unique to only you. As with all relationships, you can experience growth, friendship, arguments and distance.

According to Mindfulness coach and psychologist, Maria Hunt, "we are more likely to achieve our life-enhancing wellness goals when we develop a *cooperative* relationship between our mind and body and their sometimes-conflicting needs, one that cultivates Focus and Fitness."

Our whole life is intertwined with our very being. Though work, family, and social life may seem separate when viewed from a distance, they are all a very real and immediate part of us and our lifestyle. They provide us with our environments, interactive relationships of give and take, a sense of purpose, fulfillment, stresses, time constraints and deadlines, love and friendship, disagreements, and everything else that is our life.

1. BECOME AWARE OF YOUR THOUGHTS AND WORDS. ARE THEY LIMITING YOU? OR ARE THEY SERVING YOU?

There is one foundational secret to success in achieving breakthroughs: Your brain won't make you a liar. It will align your thoughts & speech to help your body produce exactly what you thought and spoke. Let me show you this concept in action.

My son, David, and I, work out regularly together. I asked him one day how many times he could flip the 300 lb. tractor tire. He thought about it and said, "Four". David is an athlete, strong and quite capable. He flipped the tire four times and was spent, both physically and emotionally.

The next time we flipped tires, David decided he didn't know how many times he could flip, so let's see! When he lifted the restrictions he placed on himself, he flipped many more. David Justice is now unstoppable, because he expanded his thinking and allowed his mind/body relationship to grow with the simple words, "Let's see what I can do!"

Your mind/body bottom line: You don't know what you are capable of until you try. Listen to your thoughts and words and adjust them by making them playfully open-ended. What we think and speak becomes our reality. Your mind/body relationship will help you or hinder you in your quest for a Total Body Breakthrough. Becoming aware of your thinking and speaking will help you to build a better relationship between your mind and body.

2. KNOW WHO YOU ARE

Who are you? We are not static beings. We have experiences every day that we are alive. We can be whoever and do whatever we want at any given time, with few exceptions.

What are your beliefs about your body, your health, "acting your age", your capabilities, your needs and desires, food, time, money, freedom? Have you bought into the myths of "old age"? Do you have a list of things you are not "good" at?

Your identity is who you believe yourself to be. You may have accepted someone else's perspective of you, never questioned it, and adopted it as your own. Perhaps someone told you often when you were younger that you were no good at sports, and you spent your life believing this, never attempting any physical activities. Or perhaps you came up with an interpretation on your own, such as when you noticed that you had to "work" at something that came easily to someone else – by being "a comparing creature," in other words.

Is your identity tied to your weight, a disability, a perceived weakness, your body shape, your expertise, your job, your sport, your family, your personality, your smile, or your hair color?

What would happen to your identity if any of those factors change? If you have tied your identity to something that no longer is, you may feel you no longer know who you are. You are who you are or who you let others (or your own unbalanced beliefs) dictate who you are (which limits what you can do and become).

Your mind/body bottom line: You are not your weight; you are not your medals and diplomas. Those are what you look like and what you've done. You are not the same person you were last year. You have retained some of your foundational beliefs. Are they helping or hurting you? Which ones do you want to feed?

3. LISTEN TO YOUR BODY

Your body talks to you in many different ways. From the moment you awaken until you fall asleep, it speaks to you with emotion, physical sensations, memories, and urges to action (or inaction).

If you are carrying excess weight on your body, your knees (designed for your average size body) are now being taxed with excessive force and being made to move under duress. They creak and groan, they complain and protest as their cartilage and surface structures wear away under that pressure and strain. They send pain signals through your body to your mind, screaming, STOP!

You can choose to sit and limit your movement because your knees hurt or you can choose to lose the weight your knees are complaining about.

A client with a shoulder that was pretty much immobile acknowledged holding her purse on the right for most of her life (she's in her mid 80s), then years later replaced her purse with a cane in that hand. Continued unconscious "holding" of her arm ensured that the muscles, joints, and tendons would also stay immobile. After weeks of exercise her shoulder was freed up. She had to relearn how to move the arm without shrugging her shoulder, and lose the tendency to "protect" it.

Become aware of what your body is telling you. You can compensate for it or you can do something that will create a more natural, pleasing, and long lasting result for you.

Your mind/body bottom line: What is your body saying to you? Are you listening to it? Are you responding proactively?

4. PAY ATTENTION TO YOUR OWN EXPERIENCE, YOUR OWN REALITY, THIS VERY MOMENT

Eleanor Roosevelt once said, "No one can make you feel inferior without your consent." You may not be able to control the experience of your emotions in the moment, but you can explore your feelings or bring another emotion to the forefront of your awareness.

I had a client who broke her arm in 35 places and her doctor told her she would never regain full use of that arm. I disagreed. She could have taken the doctor at his word and simply given up. She chose instead to work with me and now has full use of her arm.

Nothing in life is ever as it was. Time and circumstances change everything, sometimes for the better, sometimes not. We can embrace this moment or cling to the past, move forward, or surrender.

You wouldn't drive a car with your eyes closed. When you walk down an icy, snow covered slope, or use power tools, where is your focus? Lost in the joy of a hobby or activity you love, time just flies by. Your focus and concentration is on the task at hand. When we focus on something we make progress, we learn, we get somewhere.

Whatever we do consistently is called practice or habit. Repetition is how we learned to write, ride a bike, drive, play a sport, and all the other things we do well or regularly. Practice is a conscious effort at duplicating something. Habit is an unconscious action that once served a purpose for us that may or may not produce the same benefit we felt when we started it. Turning the light off when you leave a room is a habit that still serves a purpose.

The more we sit on a couch, the better we get at it. The more we go outside and play, the better we get at it. The more we listen to our words, our bodies, and our thoughts, the better we get at it.

Your mind/body bottom line: Become aware of what you are "practicing". It will become a part of your lifestyle very fast. Line up your thoughts, words, and actions with your objectives for your Total Body Breakthrough and things will fall into place for you more quickly.

5. THE INEVITABLE CONSEQUENCES OF ACTION AND INACTION

Your body has specific needs to regain and retain its health. You as a person have specific needs that nurture your mental, emotional, and physical health.

Developing your mind/body relationship will help you bring balance to your plan of action, and savor the moments that will bring you closer to your desires.

If you do not give your body the fresh air, sunshine, water, regular exercise, proper nutrition, sleep, and stress reduction it needs to stay healthy, your health will deteriorate. A fresh egg, dropped on a concrete floor, will break. If we don't proactively make healthy choices for our body, our body will decide our health status for us based on the tools we give it, or don't.

There are so many types of exercise and so many different flavors and textures of natural, healthy food available. Explore them, you WILL find something you like and will stick with. Whichever exercise method you choose, your body will respond. Regular exercise and proper nutrition will be your friend, if you let them.

Your mind/body bottom line: Find the healthy lifestyle activities that work for you and do them. When you find what works for you, you will stick with it. You can easily make time for things you love in your life – making time for health is easier when you discover the methods you enjoy.

6. WHERE IS YOUR FINISH LINE?

Margie participated in a transformation program and succeeded in looking great for her wedding, then life got busy, and the kids came. 12 years, 47 lbs. and 2 daily prescriptions later, Margie decided to do another transformation program. Her plan: this program would be her jump-start to regain her health and set her on track to a lifetime of good health.

For a future Olympian, the finish line is the gold medal podium, not simply getting to the Olympics, or being first at the finish line. It is standing on that podium with gold medal held high and that rush of recognition that they are the best in the world.

For many of us who are not world class athletes, the finish line is the end of a long, healthy, and prosperous life, free of disability and chronic illness with all of our faculties intact. For others, it's the class reunion or a family wedding to get into shape for, with no thought for the years to follow.

Health and fitness is a lifelong journey. One tank of gas will only get you as far as one tank of gas. Likewise, you must provide your body with proper nutrition and regular exercise as part of your everyday life for the rest of your life in order to see continued health and fitness benefits.

Your mind/body bottom line: How far out is your finish line? Is this Total Body Breakthrough a jump-start to the next mile marker? When we are a work in progress and have something to strive for, our mind/body relationship tends to cooperate for success.

7. DOES YOUR REALITY SUPPORT YOUR POSSIBILITIES?

Your Mind/Body relationship grows or stagnates through your thoughts, words, and actions. Your identity is tightly woven into your mind and body. The key to refining your reality is to discover what you truly want, enjoy and will stick with, knowing where your finish line is, and knowing that you are capable of more. A vibrant and healthy reality is there for you, should you choose to accept it.

When you practice healthy lifestyles, you will become healthier. When you practice thinking with possibilities, almost all things become possible. When you speak hopefully, positively, and confidently, your posture, stature, and thinking becomes empowering.

- Grab hold of the very basic truths in this book and find a way to make them work for you.
- Write down your objectives, keep them visible. Journal so you can see how you are progressing.
- Make the time for the activities you know will help you get where you want to go, schedule them.

Very few of us are self-motivated in every area of our lives. Find that buddy who will help hold you accountable to your plan of action, encourage you, support and celebrate your achievements, no matter how small.

*Your mind/body bottom line: You have a natural mind/body relationship that can help you succeed in your **Total Body Breakthrough**. Work with it, stay with it. You can learn to be your own best friend and use your mind/body experience to achieve more of what you want. Make a difference in your mind, and you'll make a difference in your body.*

"Training veteran Greg Justice didn't just get in on the leading edge of an emerging industry 20-some years ago, he helped create it. Opening the first personal training studio in Kansas City, Justice has, over the years, laid the groundwork for countless others to follow.

Being a trailblazer, however, takes a willingness to plow into the thicket of uncertainty. It means forging ahead with nothing but faith. As one of the true leaders of the personal training industry, Justice now has the benefit of hindsight and the insight of experience, both of which he eagerly offers up to the hundreds of trainers he has mentored."

~ Shelby Murphy,
Personal Fitness Professional magazine, *Journey to Success*, May 2009

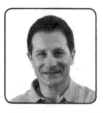

ABOUT GREG

Greg Justice, MA owner of AYC Health & Fitness, Kansas City's Original Personal Training Center, has personally trained more than 45,000 one-on-one sessions. Today, AYC specializes in corporate wellness/fitness, athletic conditioning, personal training and mindfulness coaching.

He has been actively involved in the fitness industry for more than a quarter of a century as a club manager, owner, personal fitness trainer, coach, adjunct professor, and corporate wellness supervisor. Author of "8.5 Lies & Myths About Corporate Wellness" and numerous fitness columns, Greg's corporate programs have been showcased on FOX News and in the New York Times, Fitness Business News, and many other industry publications. He currently serves at the President of the Association of Professional Personal Trainers (APPT).

He mentors and instructs trainers around the world in Corporate Wellness & Fitness. Greg Justice's Corporate Boot Camp System fills the need of CEOs and HR Professionals for achieving a means of positive, effective, and lasting change toward more healthy and productive employees. This tested and proven system combines all three major areas that businesses need to address if they are to see a healthy return on their employee benefits investment.

To learn more about Greg Justice, Corporate Fitness Expert, and receive his free Special Report "How to Implement Effective Corporate Fitness into Any Workplace", visit: www.aycfit.com.

CHAPTER 16

TIME MANAGEMENT AND A HEALTHY LIFESTYLE

BY NICK BERRY

I try to treat time like my most valuable currency. How I use my time is my 'investment' of that currency. Just like with any investment, I'm looking for a return of some type. If I invest that time well, I should be rewarded, either with more time, or with another means of fulfillment, or maybe both. If I invest it poorly, chances are that I won't find much of a return. In fact, not only could I have wasted the time I invested, I may find that I've cost myself additional time, and instead of some means of fulfillment, I'm looking at the opposite (stress, anxiety, and the issues that accompany them).

Here's an example of an investment of time that would have both a return of time as well as possible financial returns. A small business owner hires a new administrative assistant. The owner has two options with regards to training the new assistant. He can allot a certain amount of time to prepare a job description, task and responsibility list, and then train the assistant on each of the new responsibilities to make sure they are empowered to handle the responsibilities. In taking this avenue and committing the extra time up front, he could expect that the assistant should be reasonably prepared to handle most everything that he trained her to do from that point. It may have cost him a few extra hours initially, but that investment of his time should save him several times that many hours in the long run.

The alternative option is that he welcomes the assistant to work, shows her where her new desk is, and then offers, "I'm going to be pretty busy today, so I just need you to answer the phone and let me know if there are any major issues that require immediate attention." The phone rings all day, she has to interrupt the owner a few times, but at the end of the day she doesn't know anymore about how to do her job than she did at the beginning. So the cycle repeats the next day. And the next. She's unhappy because she's not learning much, and quite a few of the customers are unhappy because they couldn't be taken care of like they had hoped. The interruptions will keep going on until she is equipped with the training to handle all of the customers, ...or until she quits, ...or the customers are all frustrated and gone.

In this instance, the time he saved on the first day by not training his new assistant has now been far outweighed by the numerous ongoing interruptions to put out another fire, in addition to the stress levels for each of them (including the customers), and the financial backlash of customers leaving not to return.

Here's another example of how time can be invested: when writing a book, would you be a more efficient writer working for 2 hours with the television on, answering the phone, returning emails every couple of minutes? Or should you turn everything off, 'put the blinders on', focus and write for 45 minutes. Take a 15 minute break to check important emails and return important phone calls – but promptly put the blinders back on at the end of the 15 minutes for another 45 minute productive session? Of course it depends somewhat on how high a priority these things are, but the message is clear.

So how does your ability to focus without distraction and write a book, or your time invested to train a new assistant, tie back into a healthier you?

First of all the obvious: you get more accomplished. Being efficient and managing your time well often gives the feeling of success, and this can spill over into other areas of life and improve the quality there as well. Think big picture here though. It's not just about being able to get that book finished. It's about getting it done efficiently, and then being able to take full advantage of having done so. To use the investment analogy again, if I focus and manage to finish that 2 hour block of writing 20 minutes before I originally thought I might, I've earned that 20 minutes to invest in something else. It may be that I choose to invest it in another task or project. As long as I don't waste it, I can invest my time where I see fit, in work or my personal life. It may mean that I finish up my work-day 20 minutes early and that's additional time I've earned to spend with my wife. On the contrary, if I spoil that time, or if I make 10 minute tasks take 20 minutes, I'm stealing away that time I could potentially invest.

It's important to note here the meaning where I used the phrase 'finished'. I mean finished correctly, not temporarily. Among many famous John Wooden quotes is, "If you don't have time to do it right, when will you have time to do it again?" The importance of making sure a task is done properly is not to be overlooked. Being 'finished working' is not the same as having 'work finished'.

It's no secret that effective time management helps you get more done each day. What many fail to recognize though are the positive effects that getting more done can have on your health, or to counter that, what negative effects getting less done can have on your health. Poor time management leads to that 'lost' feeling, running around 'like a chicken with your head cut off', putting out fires, scrambling all day and getting nothing accomplished. Those feelings can quickly turn into health issues:

- Stress. High blood pressure, anxiety, heart disease. Chronic stress can slow digestion, raise heart rates, increase insulin levels.
- Loss of sleep. Sleep is necessary for the brain to perform optimally. Without adequate sleep, you are more prone to stress, making it more difficult to focus on important goals and tasks.
- Lower stamina.

All of these items contribute to a lower self-esteem and lowered work performance, in addition to detracting from your quality of life even in the areas of life you enjoy most. Maybe it's your job, family, faith, hobby – that eventually is affected.

TIPS TO MANAGE TIME EFFECTIVELY

We're not all born with excellent time management skills. Here are some rules that I use to manage my time, and have clients apply to manage theirs as well. They work if you hold yourself accountable to them. With our business coaching clients who are working on time management, I tell them to treat themselves like an employee with these rules. If you wouldn't let an employee break this rule, don't let yourself break it.

- **Be prompt for everything.** To me, this is the most effective practice in good time management, and it becomes habitual. People who are prompt tend to be efficient. You'll also find that those who can't be prompt even for minor commitments probably can't be prompt for major ones either. Being prompt shows a respect for your time, as well as for those who are sharing that time with you. And being late shows a lack of respect for each party's time. You may want to implement a '5 minutes early is 10 minutes late' (or 2 minutes early is 3 minutes late') rule for yourself, to begin creating that habit of promptness.
- **Set a schedule and take pride in being able to stick to it.** Plan each day ahead of time. Planning your day can help you accomplish more and feel more in control of your life. Write a to-do list, putting the most important tasks at the top. Unfortunately, things are going to pop up out of nowhere. Having a schedule you can stick to helps you manage those unforeseen items most effectively, and without feeling overwhelmed. You'll see that as you get better at planning out days, then planning weeks and months gets much less daunting. And it's important you take pride in adhering to the schedule, in order to maintain accountability.
- **Don't let 10 minute tasks take 20 minutes.** Or even 15. Set appropriate deadlines and stick to them. Again, this will become habitual, and you'll begin to take pride in completing tasks on time. Then you'll start earning more time to reinvest as you see fit. You'll also see less 'do-overs' on tasks you may not have completed entirely in the past.
- **Bill yourself.** This is an exercise that I began doing to evaluate how I was spending my time. Keep a log of everything you do for every minute of an entire day (or more if needed), as if you were going to bill yourself for the time spent on tasks. You've got to be honest with yourself. If you started on a task at 1:00, and finished at 1:18, but you stared out the window for

5 minutes in between, you didn't really work for 18 minutes, did you? At the end of the day, you'll see a lot of blocks under 10 minutes that you can't account for anything productive happening. Those small gaps add up to a lot of time you could make a better investment with. This leads us to another rule....

- **Fill small gaps with small tasks.** If you've got 10 minutes between phone calls, find something small you can complete or work on in 10 minutes. That's not daydream time, nor is it time for ESPN.com. Could you catch up on reading? Schedule a Dr.'s appointment? Get a couple of bills in the mail? Find a receipt you needed? File some of the papers stacked on your desk?

Other tips to manage your time:

- **Say no to nonessential tasks.** Consider your goals and schedule before agreeing to take on additional work. You may have to delegate. Take a look at your to-do list and consider what you can pass on to someone else or just isn't your highest priority.
- **Take the time you need to do a quality job.** Doing work right the first time may take more time upfront, but errors usually result in time spent making corrections, which takes more time overall.
- **Break large, time-consuming tasks into smaller tasks.** Work on them a few minutes at a time until you get them all done.
- **Dreaded Tasks.** Work on a dreaded task for a set amount of time each day. You'll get better at finishing them, instead of trying to find reasons not to do them.
- **Get plenty of sleep, have a healthy diet and exercise regularly.** A healthy lifestyle can improve your focus and concentration, which will help improve your efficiency so that you can complete your work in less time.
- **Take a break when needed.** Too much stress can derail your attempts at getting organized. When you need a break, take one. Take a walk. Do some quick stretches at your workstation. Take a day of vacation to rest and re-energize.
- **Prioritize.** See what needs to be done, then do the most important first.
  - o Make sure the activities include something that takes you towards your goals. If not, why are you doing it?

o   Recognize the difference between what you
    NEED vs. WANT.

As with any attempt at creating a better habit, you can't implement all of these practices overnight. Pick one or two that really seem to resonate with you and run with it. Then add another as you get better. You'll see that they all start to work together and can become second nature to you.

Here's a valuable story I was once told about how to go about implementing time management:

A time management expert was speaking to a group of business students, and decided to use an illustration.

He told them they were having a quiz. He took a large jar and placed it on the table in the front of the room. Then he took out some golf ball-sized rocks and began placing them in the jar.

When the jar was filled to the top and no more rocks would fit inside, he asked, "Is this jar full?" Everyone replied, "Yes."

He then pulled out a bucket of smaller rocks, near the size of peas. He dumped some of the smaller rocks in and shook the jar so the smaller pieces would settle into the spaces between the larger rocks. He then asked the group once more, "Is the jar full?"

"Probably not," one of them answered.

"Good!" he replied. Then he pulled out a bucket of sand, and started pouring it into the jar with the rocks. The sand filled all of the spaces left between the rocks and the gravel. Then he again asked, "Is this jar full?" "No!" the class shouted.

Once again he said, "Good." Then he took a pitcher of water and poured into the jar, filling it completely to the top. Then he asked the class, "What is the point of this illustration?"

Someone said, "The point is, no matter how full your schedule is, if you try really hard you can always fit some more things in it!"

"No," the speaker replied, "that's not the point. The truth that this illustration teaches us is: If you don't put the big rocks in first, you'll never get them in at all."

That story illustrates perfectly how important it is to prioritize, and to prioritize you have to understand the difference in what you need vs. what you want. Make the decision to manage your time better, and you will be consistently rewarded with lower stress levels and feelings of accomplishment, and therefore a healthier lifestyle.

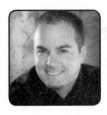

ABOUT NICK

Nick Berry has spent his entire career as an Entrepreneur. His experience has given him the opportunity to become a Business Coach and Consultant, allowing him to help thousands of other small business owners, both in and out of the fitness industry.

Currently, Nick has helped build and co-owns the International Youth Conditioning Association, The Athletic Revolution International youth fitness franchise, the marketing and consulting companies Fitness Consulting Group and Ultimate Business Systems, which he partners with Pat Rigsby, Facility Formula, and multiple other fitness businesses, including a health club in Owensboro, Ky.

CHAPTER 17

THE MIND: UNDERSTAND THE GREAT POWER WITHIN YOU

– UNDERSTANDING PRECEDES CHANGE

BY JUSTIN YULE

B efore we can make changes, we must understand what controls them – *the mind*.

The mind is governed by specific, universal laws, even if we ignore them. Consider gravity. Imagine yourself on the top of a building, deciding to step off the edge. Gravity dictates that you will fall to the ground, no exceptions, with potentially dire consequences. Ignorance of the law does not change the result. Similar laws govern our universe. Get familiar with these laws and work in harmony with them, or ignore them and pay the price.

The Great Law – *Energy Is*

Elementary science class taught that all things are made up of the same kind of energy. Look at your hand. It's a mass of molecules vibrating at a very high rate of speed. The chair you are sitting on, the book you are reading, the water you drink, and the food you eat are all made up of the same energy. This law tells us that everything that ever was, is, or will be has always existed in some form.

The ability for planes to fly has always existed. It took the imagination, will, and determination of the Wright brothers to prove it.

Not long ago, the concept of typing a few keywords into a search engine on the Internet to instantly retrieve millions of information resources sounded absurd. Today, people access the Internet from home computers and devices that fit in the palm of a hand. The laws that made this possible have always existed. We just needed awareness to bring them about.

The same rules apply to physical health and fitness. It just takes an awareness of key information and a willingness to abide by certain laws. Tapping this energy allows us to do virtually anything.

I believe Bob Proctor is one of today's greatest mentors. Most of the information here comes from the Life Success programs and seminars I've been fortunate enough to participate in. Since "tapping into Bob's energy" and raising my awareness through his teaching, along with other great mentors and leaders, I've personally been able to bring about extraordinarily positive changes in my life. I know the lessons in this book will do the same for you.

The **Law of Vibration** states that everything vibrates and nothing rests. Conscious awareness of this vibration is called *feeling*. Your thoughts control your vibration and paradigms. Paradigms are essentially a multitude of habits developed by your perception, your view of the world. For example, maybe your mother is obese and you look a lot like her. Then, you assume that you will be obese and you cannot see yourself any other way. Therefore, the actions that you take (or don't take) cause you to be obese. The result reinforces the paradigm and the vicious cycle continues.

What can you do? Replace your negative thoughts with something positive from outside that paradigm, and hold that image to block out negative thoughts. Choose to think and feel positive and successful. Until your thoughts shift to a more pure and healthy image, you will never be able to have the fitness success you desire.

RATES OF VIBRATION

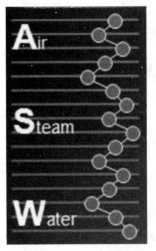

Water is energy vibrating at a specific rate. Heating the water increases the rate of vibration. When it reaches 212°F (100°C), water boils. As water continues to heat, it gradually changes to steam and to air. It is still the same energy. Each level of vibration is connected to the one directly above and directly below it. Water, steam and air are the same energy, vibrating at different speeds on specific frequencies.

This simple concept has deeper meaning in relation to human potential.

LEVELS OF EXISTENCE

We are spiritual beings living in physical bodies. Let's refer to our spiritual level of existence as energy.

We have also been gifted with intellect, which includes imagination, memory, perception, will, reason, and intuition. We can use our intellectual factors to tap into our spirit and improve the results in our physical world.

IMAGINATION: "The faculty of imagining, or of forming mental images or concepts of what is not actually present to the senses." [1]

Your imagination can build beautiful mental images that literally create the world around you. Everything is created twice, first in the imagination and second in the physical world. Imagination gives us the power of visualization to achieve physical results; it is a critical component to success.

MEMORY: "The mental capacity or faculty of retaining and reviving facts, events, impressions, etc., or of recalling or recognizing previous experiences."[2]

There is no such thing as a bad memory, only underdeveloped memory.

---

1 http://dictionary.reference.com/browse/imagination
2 http://dictionary.reference.com/browse/memory

Memory, like muscle, becomes weak when it is underused and strong when it is properly developed.

PERCEPTION: "The act or faculty of apprehending by means of the senses or mind; cognition; understanding."[3]

Perception lets you see things differently. When you change your viewpoint, you change how things look. Perception is a powerful intellectual factor and a major contributor to the formation of paradigms. Your paradigms literally control everything you do – and your results. What you see is what you get.

WILL (WILL POWER): "The control of one's impulses and actions; self-control."[4]

Your will enables you to concentrate and hold onto an idea while excluding all obstacles and distractions. Everyone has will power, but they have it at different levels of development. When your goal fulfills a big enough *why*, you will do anything to accomplish it.

REASON: "The mental power concerned with forming conclusions, judgments, or inferences."[5]

Reason enables you to choose and originate thoughts, build and ponder ideas, accept or reject ideas. You're in charge. You determine the results!

INTUITION: "The direct perception of truth, fact, etc., independent of any reasoning process; immediate apprehension."[6]

Intuition picks up vibrations from energy and allows you to read people and situations. Intuition is the inner voice that tells you the right thing to do. Trust it.

---

3 http://dictionary.reference.com/browse/perception
4 http://dictionary.reference.com/browse/willpower
5 http://dictionary.reference.com/browse/reason
6 http://dictionary.reference.com/browse/intuition

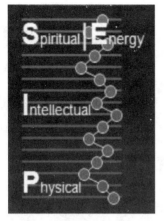

Our three levels of existence, (1) physical, (2) intellectual, and (3) spiritual/energy, occur on different frequencies or rates of vibration. However, just like the water, steam and air, they are all connected.

We can conclude that all parts, seen and unseen, are connected and spirit/energy always manifests itself in a physical form. You may not be able to see gravity or air, but they exist. You may not see yourself in a beautiful, healthy body, but it exists. Tap into your mind to move from spiritual to physical existence. When you understand how your mind works and can tap into your spirit, you will manifest the healthy, fit body that has always existed.

It's like the little boy who watched a sculptor create a magnificent statue from a block of marble and asked, "How did you know that guy was in there?"

UNDERSTANDING THE MIND

The mind works in pictures. Think of your car or house, and a picture immediately comes to mind. How do you picture yourself?

Dr. Thurman Fleet, founder of the Concept Theory, developed the stick-person drawing to explain how the mind works. It has three parts: the conscious mind, the subconscious mind, and the body.

Your conscious mind is your thinking mind. It determines your attitude and success, accepts or rejects ideas, and chooses your thoughts. Once your conscious mind accepts an idea, it is immediately impressed upon your subconscious mind.

Unlike your conscious mind, your subconscious mind is unable to reject ideas. It operates in accordance with an orderly law. Repeated conscious thoughts become fixed ideas until they are consciously replaced by new ideas (paradigms). You can force a paradigm shift by consciously filtering what enters your subconscious mind.

Your body is the house you live in, the physical medium that contains your mind. The consciously chosen thoughts and images that you impress upon your subconscious mind move your body into action. Actions determine results.

Imagine a child raised by obese parents who learns a sedentary lifestyle and unhealthy eating habits. Over time the child forms a fat, nonathletic paradigm. The child avoids physical activities, eats fattening foods, and gets fat. The child's reinforced paradigm leads to adult obesity. Did the child become an obese adult because of genetics or because of actions dictated by a fat, nonathletic paradigm?

The thoughts you choose create the image you hold. The image you hold controls the feelings you have. The feelings you have cause the actions you take. The actions you take control the results you get.

RAISING THE BAR – INCREASING YOUR LEVEL OF PERFORMANCE

Cybernetics is the study of control and communication in machines to regulate or reach an end goal. Essentially, a cybernetic mechanism is a device that regulates a machine to achieve an end result. Thermostats are cybernetic mechanisms that maintain consistent room temperatures. Similarly, airplanes are guided to their destinations by autopilot functions.

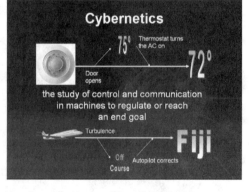

Psycho-cybernetics considers the human mechanism relevant to potential. Maxwell Maltz, author of Psycho-Cybernetics, wanted to understand why goal setting works and studied self-affirmation and visualization techniques in the mind-body connection. He specified techniques to develop a positive inner goal that achieves a positive outer goal. Inner attitudes are essential because outer success can never surpass what is visualized.

How does this apply to weight loss?

Right now you are mentally programmed (conditioned) to weigh a certain amount. You behave in a way that brings about that result. If you

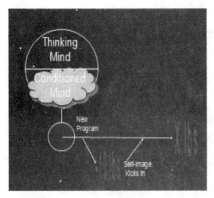

change your behavior by starting an exercise program, you will lose weight. At some point, this change will create a disturbance in your mental program, and your mind will tune into your former weight and literally halt your progress. You will change your behavior, go back to your mental program, and regain your weight. This cycle will continue *until* you see yourself at your desired weight and act to maintain it. You must change the "conditioned" mind.

Your present results are a direct reflection of your thinking at a frequency lower than the frequency of your goal. You must think and act at the same frequency as that of your goal. *Success and failure are both the offspring of thought.*

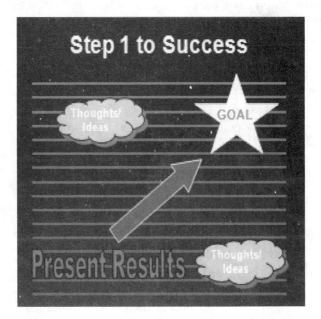

VISUALIZATION:
SEE YOURSELF ACHIEVING YOUR GOAL

Visualization is powerful. Use your imagination to picture yourself in the healthy, fit body you want. Feel it.

In a well-known study on Creative Visualization, Russian scientists compared the training schedules of four groups of Olympic athletes:

- Group 1 had 100% physical training
- Group 2 had 75% physical training with 25% mental training
- Group 3 had 50% physical training with 50% mental training
- Group 4 had 25% physical training with 75% mental training.

Group 4 performed the best. "The Soviets discovered that mental images can act as a prelude to muscular impulses."[7]

Olympic athletes use visualization to mentally prepare for competition. They rehearse exactly what they have to do to win. Sports psychologists say that visualization boosts athletes' confidence by forcing them to picture themselves winning. It also helps them concentrate on their physical moves rather than the distractions around them.[8]

VISUALIZE TO ACTUALIZE

Creative Visualization occurs in the first person, present tense, as if it is unfolding around you. Here is a visualization exercise that I have successfully used to help clients overcome weight-loss plateaus:

1. Draw a line down the center of a piece of paper.
2. On the left-hand side, write everything you dislike about your body.
3. On the right-hand side, change all the statements from the left-hand side to positive ones. Begin all statements with "I am so happy and grateful now that..." (For example, "I am so happy

---

7 Robert Scaglione, William Cummins, Karate of Okinawa: Building Warrior Spirit, Tuttle Publishing, 1993, ISBN 096264840X.

8 Fiona McCormack, "Mind games," Scholastic Scope, Vol. 54, Iss. 10, New York: Jan 23, 2006

and grateful now that I have sculpted and defined arms.")

4. Cut the paper down the center.
5. Burn the left-hand side.
6. As you watch it burn, release all your negative emotions.
7. Hang the paper with your positive affirmations where you will see it often.
8. Read each statement, and feel the joy those results will bring.
9. Picture yourself and, most importantly, imagine how good it will feel when those statements are true.
10. Only when your positive affirmations are true in your mind, can you make them true in reality.

Remember, all things are created twice - first in the imagination and second in the physical world. Start imagining exactly what you want.

ACTION ITEMS

- ❒ Complete the Self Assessment on the following page
- ❒ Read *As a Man Thinketh* by James Allen
- ❒ Read *You Were Born Rich* by Bob Proctor
- ❒ Read or listen to *The Strangest Secret* by Earl Nightingale
- ❒ Watch and read *The Secret* by Rhonda Byrne
- ❒ Read *The Power of the Subconscious Mind* by Dr. Joseph Murphy
- ❒ Read *Psycho-Cybernetics* by Maxwell Maltz
- ❒ Sign up for *Insight of the Day*, and start your days with positive messages.
- ❒ Create an affirmation statement(s) and visualize your success
  - Put your affirmation statement(s) in places where you will see them often – your bathroom mirror, car, and desk. Keep them on a card in your pocket at all times.
- ❒ Create a vision board. Cut out pictures of your goal (i.e., fit bodies, athletes, etc.) and make a collage that you can view often. See yourself, feel yourself as a positive success.

SELF-ASSESSMENT

Name: _____ Date: _____

What are paradigms? How can they help me achieve my goal?

_____

_____

How do I perceive myself?

_____

_____

How does my self-perception affect my goal?

_____

_____

How do I want to perceive myself?

_____

_____

What is my fitness goal? Why?

_____

_____

Am I worth it? _____

What can I do today to program my subconscious mind and act to achieve and maintain my goal?

_____

_____

How will I feel after I achieve my goal?

_____

_____

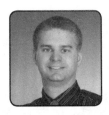

ABOUT JUSTIN

Justin Yule, BS, CPT has been studying health and fitness for 22 years, practicing as a personal trainer for the last 13 years, and has helped thousands of clients reach their fitness goals through his personal supervision and personal training management roles. Today, Justin focuses on population-based training and specializes in fitness boot camps for all levels.

Justin holds a Bachelor's degree in Physical Education with a Concentration in Adult Fitness (1997) from The State University of New York at Cortland. He is also a National Academy of Sports Medicine Certified Personal Trainer.

Justin has worked with men and women of all ages and physical abilities in his career as a personal trainer. In 2002, Justin was named the Most Valuable Trainer with Life Time Fitness. He then served multiple roles and received recognition in Management, Research & Development, and Education at the local and national level.

In 2009, Justin authored his first book, *The Science of Getting Fit*, and launched his own weight loss and fitness boot camp program, Look Great at the Lake Boot Camp.

Something most people don't realize about Justin is that he has struggled with weight his whole life. Being in shape is something Justin has to work on daily. Being a former 'fat kid', he understands the stresses and difficulties that come with being overweight and out of shape. With his experience and education, Justin has developed a sound weight loss and fitness program – with proven results.

Justin has a simple philosophy when it comes to health, fitness and life in general: Have Faith and Take Action! He feels that most people who lose at anything focus on the negativity of the tasks while those who win simply focus on the end result.

Justin's goal is to offer health and fitness solutions for busy men and women by providing them with efficient and effective programs that are both safe and fun. His boot camp program is available locally and online. Look Great at the Lake Boot Camp, a community based weight loss and fitness program in Chanhassen, MN, delivers the highest quality personal training program in town. Look Great at the Lake Boot Camp ONLINE, brings the best of his live program to the web; so anyone, anywhere can take advantage of his incredible results producing program.

In addition to the scientifically proven workouts, each participant receives meal plans with done-for-you recipes, a copy of Justin's book *The Science of Getting Fit*, and continuing education through daily blog posts, weekly motivational emails and monthly Q&A calls. Members are fully supported in and out of class and can communicate with each other through an online members' only forum. This attention to detail and 360-degree approach to health and fitness is what creates such a high rate of return on investment for his members.

CHAPTER 18

HOW TO MAKE FITNESS FUN! WELL, BETTER THAN FUN...TRULY REWARDING.

BY NIKI DAVIS

Does this title sound like an oxymoron? Does anyone really enjoy exercising? What if I told you fitness could not only be more fun, but it could also be rewarding on so many more levels, inspire you to work harder at your job, your relationships and even be a better parent. Now you really think I am nuts, right? Quite the contrary, I just like to take my clients fitness very seriously and as a career personal trainer, it is important to me that my clients want to exercise not just for the next 10 weeks, but for the rest of their lives.

Let me tell you a story about a lady named Lynn. Lynn came to me about 7 years ago after I had worked with her son over the summer between his junior and senior year of high school so that he could make it onto the varsity crew team. He had worked hard all summer and did indeed make it onto the varsity team. Was he having fun during those one-on-one sessions as I worked him harder and harder and with less and less rest and then sent him for a run when we were finished? I would like to think so, but in the moment, I doubt he did. Did he enjoy himself when he was finishing first or second on conditioning runs instead of close to last like in the previous season's tryouts? You bet he did!

Let's get back to Lynn, as I said she came to me that Fall and decided that she would like to start exercising more regularly and thought I could help her get more fit. So we sat down, set some goals and started to exercise. Before long, she was a regular client twice a week with me. But the tide really changed when Lynn decided to take me up on competing in a triathlon in the spring and she joined my beginner triathlon class. We had from that Fall all the way until Mother's Day in May, plenty of time, I assured her, to train for the big day, …and so we began. Now Lynn wasn't just exercising, she was training for an event! Suddenly, she was coming into the gym on days that we weren't scheduled to meet. She was working on her swim, running on the treadmill and meeting our group for bike rides on the weekend. Did I mention that Lynn was at that time mother to 3 teenagers, on the fundraising board for the crew team, and busy with a million other things that involved taking care of everyone else. But suddenly she was taking 3-4 hours a week to focus on herself.

When Mother's Day came, she was ready. She was a bit nervous, but confident and ready. Lynn finished the triathlon, a women's only event where the tables were turned. For a change, her husband and 3 children were there to support her, cheer her on and had tears in their eyes when she finished. I was so proud of her as she crossed the finish line, as was her family. However, the icing on the cake for me was finding out months later that her teenage daughter had a picture of Lynn, her mother, finishing her triathlon on her computer as a screen saver. Do you think this sent a message to her two daughters?

There is a direct correlation between your physical sense of self and your self-esteem. If you feel more comfortable in your skin, it will show. You will carry yourself differently. Furthermore, they say children get most of their self-esteem from their same-sex parent. So, do we as women want to teach our daughters that once you have children you don't take care of yourself anymore, and just do for everyone else? Do men want to teach their sons physical fitness and sports are only for the youth. …Then on to 60 hour work weeks?

When was the last time you challenged yourself to do something that you really didn't think you could do? I mean physically. Lynn didn't know how to swim properly, hadn't biked in years and never for 12 miles, and running wasn't exactly her favorite pastime. The reason it scares us so much is that we are afraid to fail, but what if you could overcome that fear, ... prepare, train, succeed. I guarantee this new-found success will carry over into other aspects of your life.

Let me tell you something else, I think the more daunting the goal seems to someone, the more the total impact across the board when you realize you can succeed and conquer . Reminding yourself or even learning for the first time that you are stronger than you think, and can push through obstacles and road blocks, can be profound. Then you apply this discovery, this same logic to work, and no job opening is above you, no account too big to handle.

You set goals, get a coach, build a support team, get the right equipment and, one step at a time, you reach those finish lines too. This wasn't an ultimate Ironman that Lynn completed. It was a 1/4 mile swim, 12 mile bike course and 2 mile run, but how many of you think "I could never do that"? Let me tell you, you can, and if you do, you won't be the same after.

I am not saying everyone should be a triathlete, but you should try something new, and through the coming years as you explore exercise you should continue to try new things. Our bodies were built with muscles to be used, and humans were meant to interact. Yet we spend more and more time motionless in seated positions, and less time face-to-face with other people. So, what do you want to do about it?

Below are 9 Keys to workout success and to set the stage for enjoying a rewarding exercise program:-

1. **TAKE MEASUREMENTS AND SET GOALS** – Ok, I admit taking measurements doesn't sound like much fun. In fact, this thought is enough to scare some people away from starting at all, but how will you know how far you have come, or when to celebrate your victories if you don't know where you started?. I recommend taking at least body weight, circumference and body fat percentage measurements. If you haven't exercised in years, I also recommend you go get some blood work done. Again, more for the fun and reward later of seeing how much

better your Cholesterol, blood pressure and blood sugar will be, once you are exercising regularly.

Goals are equally important and should be as specific as possible and include a goal date. " I would like to lose twenty pounds by my 35th birthday, May 29, 2011" is much more powerful and likely to be met than a vague goal like, "I would like to lose some weight" or "I would like to tone up." What exactly does that mean? How much weight? By when? How do you know when you have reached "tone up"? Ideally, set and re-evaluate these goals at least quarterly, so every three months you have goals to focus on. I usually have my clients set 3 different types of goals.

- **End Result Goals** – This is the one people usually have no trouble coming up with. "I want to lose 20 pounds", "I want to wear a size 6" for women or "I want to fit back into size 36 pants" for men.
- **Process Goals** – This is where most people miss setting a goal. The Process should be a separate goal. How do you plan to accomplish the End Result goal? "I am going to exercise 4-6 days a week for the next 3 months", "I am going to stop drinking Soda/start eating breakfast", and "I will take a yoga class each week to work on my flexibility and help reduce stress"
- **Performance Goals** – Fitness isn't just about weight or pants size. So, this goal only has to do with performance. "I would like to run a mile without stopping", "I would like to do 12 pushups from my toes", "I would like to learn to rollerblade/swim/rock climb".

2. **TAKE A FRIEND OR MAKE A FRIEND** – You set your goals, and hopefully posted them where you can see them regularly, but that doesn't make training toward them fun. What about those mornings when you plan on going for a run but it's cold outside and sleeping in sounds sooooooo good. If you have a friend that you are meeting you will get up and go. If you are going to cycling class and know your classmates will wonder where you were, you will get up and go. Get to know other people at your gym, join a running club or inspire your friends

or coworkers to start exercising with you. Go for a bike ride/ try a dance class together/ sign up for adult swim lessons and then go for coffee or a smoothie instead of just meeting for another high calorie lunch.

3. **GET OUT OF YOUR COMFORT ZONE. EVEN LAUGH AT YOURSELF** – If you want to have fun you have to try something new and maybe even feel a little uncomfortable. I am not a dancer but I have taken the Zumba, a Latin dance class at my gym, I felt a little silly and uncoordinated but I had fun. When I took Group Kick, our version of a Kick Boxing class, I really felt strong and like I could "kick some butt", but I think the only butt that was kicked was mine – from all those kicks and jumps in class. Trying new things will spice up your exercise and help it to be anything but routine, and you might just find that you really enjoy doing something you hadn't expected.

4. **COMPETE!** – 5K, triathlon, dodge ball, basketball league. It doesn't matter if you were formerly an athlete or not. Some of us really thrive on competition, and tapping into this can make the difference to a lasting exercise regimen. Competing with others in your age group or competing to beat yourself can serve as serious motivation. One year my fitness goal was to beat the time of the only 1/2 marathon I had completed before having my two boys. I did it , it was my little competition with my former self to prove to no one but myself that I was as fit as I had been before I had the kids, and it felt great!

5. **TRAIN VS. EXERCISE** – Just like Lynn, when you are training for something, your workouts have direction. You no longer wander aimlessly into the gym just to see what cardio machines are open. If you are training for a marathon, you are usually running at least 3 days a week with longer progressive runs once a week. There is no guessing, you are following a training regimen. Bonus, the event itself serves as the end date of your goal.

6. **BE A PART OF SOMETHING BIGGER THAN YOURSELF** – Sign up for an event that raises money for a cause. Check out: www.teamintraining.com, www.nationalmssociety.org, www.tour.diabetes.org or www.avonwalk.org to name only a few. There are a myriad events out there, catering to from first timers to elite athletes, that not only include team training

and coaching, but keep you inspired – as you train with and for people who need your support. Many of these events are not races either, so if competing doesn't appeal to you, try the Avon walk for breast cancer or the 2-day 150 mile bike ride for Muscular Sclerosis. Also, many companies will match fundraising, so check with your employer and see if they have a matching program. Then gather some coworkers together for some true team building!

7. **MOVE EVERY DAY** – give yourself credit for increasing even your non-exercise activity. Wear a pedometer! This is a great experiment and an easy thing to start. Buy yourself a pedometer and track how many steps you take per day. I work on my feet and on a typical workday, before I do any exercise for myself, I take between 12,000-15,000 steps. However, I have a client that tele-commutes and works from home on a computer. I was shocked to find out that on a day that he doesn't exercise he was regularly logging only 1,000-1,800 steps per day. I couldn't believe it! This kind of inactivity can stall even the best efforts to get in shape. The American Heart Association recommends 10,000 steps a day. Research shows that the average American takes 2,000-5,000 "lifestyle steps", just going about their regular day. By adding just 30 minutes of walking or jogging per day you can raise this number to 10,000 steps. I wore a pedometer consistently for months because of a program we had at work, and you might be surprised how simple yet motivating and telling it is to see the actual #'s every day. Then when you realize that we can all be extremely inactive at times, you might find yourself washing your own car, walking the dog a little further, or playing tag with the kids instead of just watching. Every step counts!

8. **HIRE A PROFESSIONAL!** – Many people think that trainers only have clients that see them 2-3 times a week. Take it from me, yes, I have those clients but I also have some clients I see once a month, once a quarter or every once in a while. If you are ready to take your training to the next level treat yourself to a personal training session every once in a while. If I have someone I know is seeing me to set up a workout plan that they can carry out on their own, I approach the sessions a little

differently. I try to educate them on why I put certain exercises in the program by explaining concepts and specific exercise form concerns. I use the fantasy football analogy often, if you were making your own team, you would research credentials, hire proven coaches and recruit quality teammates. The same is true here, find a trainer, nutritionist and support team that will ensure your success.

9. **SPEAK POSITIVELY ABOUT EXERCISE** – This might sound silly to some, but if you dread exercise or look at it as a punishment for over-indulgence, then of course it isn't going to be fun. Change your internal feelings and dialog about exercise. "I am going to take the 6:00 pm Yoga class on Fridays because it always helps me decompress after a long work week.", "I feel so much stronger since I have been lifting weights." or "Fall is such a beautiful time to go out and hike." This small change can have a big impact on how we view and think about exercise. Try it!

Set Goals, Track your progress, build your team, train for an event, and succeed! Get in touch with your physical self and start to enjoy exercising maybe for the first time in a long time, or for the first time ever!

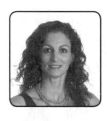

ABOUT NIKI

Niki Davis' Qualifications:

Bachelor Of Science-University of Florida-Exercise and Sport Sciences

NASM-Performance Enhancement Specialist

ACSM-Health Fitness Instructor

NSCA-Certified Strength and Conditioning Specialist

Triathlon coach and pre/post natal training instructor

Niki Davis has been sharing her passion for exercise through personal training and coaching for the last 13 years. She truly believes in changing and improving quality of life though fitness. For the last 10 years she has been working at the RDV Sportsplex Athletic Club in Orlando, Florida. A 365,000 square foot state-of-the-art facility . Her clientele includes teenagers, expectant moms, competitive triathletes and runners, as well as first-time exercisers and seniors. In addition to training at the RDV Sportsplex, she also coordinates their new member orientation program and continuing education for the RDV Sportsplex Fitness staff.

Niki has represented the RDV Sportsplex as a fitness expert on local TV "Fitness Tip" spots for Fox 35 News, and on the radio show 'The Philips File' on 104.1 FM.

Niki herself is a competitive age group triathlete, avid runner, yoga instructor, wife and mother of two very active boys!

To contact Niki Davis, check out: www.rdvsportsplex.com or more directly at: www.ndavis@rdvsportsplex.com 407-916-2543 or loveyourfitness@gmail.com

Niki Davis-Personal Trainer, Performance Coach & Exercise Enthusist

CHAPTER 19

GETTING BETTER WITH BANDS!!

– A RESISTANCE BAND TRAINING TRANSFORMATION

BY DAVE SCHMITZ, THE BAND MAN

t was 1997 and I was 34 years young and from a mirror perspective in pretty good shape. I was hitting the gym five to six days a week doing the traditional chest and back routine on Monday, shoulders and arms on Tuesdays, legs on Wednesdays and light cardio on Thursdays. I was a self-proclaimed gym rat that loved lifting weights and working out. I also loved athletics but had not been competitive for the past six years. After 15 years of pumping iron I found myself extremely stiff, suffering from chronic shoulder irritation as well as lower back and elbow stiffness that periodically fell into the pain category which limited my workout! Yes, looking good in my mid 30's was important but when you can't run very well, can't throw a ball without your shoulder feeling like it was about to fall off, and your two grade school children are starting to kick your butt in a simple game of kickball, there is something wrong with this picture. Not to mention, my professional career was as an orthopedic physical therapist that was successfully built on getting patients with these very same problems better. Talk about 'the pot calling the kettle black'. Here I was instructing people on a daily basis about working consistently on flexibility, full range-of-motion exercises, and multi-directional strength training while I went back into the gym to beat up my body doing the exact opposite: minimal stretching, all straight plane movements, and essentially the same muscle-head workout every Monday, Wednesday and Friday.

On a beautiful morning in June, 1997 I made the decision I was going to start doing some sprint training workouts. So I went out, warmed up like I knew I had to, and proceeded to start doing some 50 yard sprints. It took only one full out sprint for my body to inform me that this was not going to happen. Not only did my hip joints and lower back feel like two solid boards, my non-flexible hamstrings strongly informed me to shut it down or they were going to blow.

After all the iron pumping, all the 5:00 am workouts, all the gut wrenching supersets, the thousands of crunches and back-killing heavy squats; I was left with a body that looked good but could not function at anything higher than a fast walk. Coming from a licensed physical therapist that loved athletics and felt he knew a lot about athletic performance, this was a real slap in the face. Something obviously had to change if I wanted to physically feel better and get back to being an athlete, not just looking the part.

Fortunately, it was during this same year that I took a trip with a good coaching friend of mine to Notre Dame University to attend a coach's football clinic. I do not coach so when they started talking X's and O's I ventured out to look around. I walked into the indoor practice facility and came across a little man going ballistic with these large, and I mean LARGE, rubber bands. He was probably the most athletic 64 year old gentleman I had ever seen. At one point, he dropped right into the splits which made my hamstrings cringe instantly.

Within about 20 minutes he was able to demonstrate to the handful of us standing there, how to run, stretch, push, pull, squat, throw, and jump using these simple rubber bands. Instantly the light went off. It was no wonder why this 64 year old ex-coach was flexible, strong, powerful, and agile. The things he was doing looked, smelled and felt athletic. At age

64 he was doing everything I could not do well at 34. Needless to say, for the next three hours I watched every move he made. To make a long story very short, I left that day armed with two rubber bands that totally changed my life physically, personally and professionally. I guess you could say I had just witnessed a major life-changing event.

FLASH FORWARD THREE YEARS

Needless to say, I wore those two bands out teaching, training and experimenting on myself as well as anyone that would listen. The level of performance I was able to recapture in myself, as well as my clients or patients, was amazing. Almost two years to the day, I was now sprinting better than I did in high school, touching the rim of the hoop and dropping spontaneously into the splits. My kids, along with a lot of my high school athletes, were struggling to keep up.

Fortunately the physical therapist in me still remained active because that was the key to me understanding how a simple resistance band could make such a big difference. If a flat continuously looped rubber band could help injured people get better, can you imagine what it could do for people like me that wanted to look good but still play the game?

Needless to say, this resistance band training thing started not only to get legs for me personally but now professionally. In just a few short years, what started out as a personal goal of recapturing my athleticism was turning into a career-changing business opportunity as well.

IT'S A RESISTANCE BAND NOT JUST A RUBBER BAND

For years, I was just like all the other millions of fitness enthusiasts, athletes, coaches, and fitness professionals when it came to my mind set about training with resistance bands. They were a rehab tool, something used in those non-sweating health club classes, the last alternative to strength training or a way to get some muscle toning. I cannot begin to tell you how many muscle-bound athletes and treadmill-worshiping fitness enthusiast's I was able to dramatically impact with training in bands. The myths about resistance-band training could not have been further from the truth. However, breaking tradition and getting people's minds out of the magazines or away from the infomercials was going to take a while to change.

The problem was that most people did not understand how the body really functioned much less how a simple rubber band could impact that function. The body is a reactor and an adaptor. It does not think when it comes to exercise or performance. It simply reacts to stresses (i.e., exercise) applied to it and overtime adapts by increasing strength, losing weight or becoming more efficient in that exercise. Ask it to push and it pushes as hard as it needs to in order to complete the goal. Ask it to jump and it jumps as far or as high as it can. Ask it to play a game and it functionally does what it has to, to perform the game. Nothing your body does physically is ever really thought out. You just do it!!

However, with an effective exercise program, you can train it to react and respond quicker, stronger and with greater efficiency. Unfortunately, sitting on a machine or lifting deadweight while comfortably lying on a bench is not going to accomplish that.

The other thing you need to know is this....Muscles are Dumb. They do not think or show emotion. They simply react by pushing, pulling, pressing or lifting with as much force as it needs to successfully achieve the goal. Lifting a pre-determined weight is not what happens in real life. Realize that training with resistance bands is not a pre-determined resistance or set direction and allows you to jump, run, push or pull just like you do in real life. Hopefully, you can understand why it's not "just a rubber band," but rather a resistance training device that trains your body to move with greater strength, speed and efficiency.

GETTING BETTER WITH BANDS

Let's face it, exercise is your best and cheapest health insurance option. Like anything, it doesn't come without a price tag, which in this case includes effort, discipline, hard work and some time. My feeling has always been that exercise does not have to consume your day but rather be a small portion of a weekly routine. The same goes for improving performance. It's not how hard you work at it one time but rather the persistence, passion and consistency of your training. Also, it helps to do what works –not what sells magazines.

Knowing how the body functions, and what it takes to effectively keep it running well, is where an exercise program needs to start. Once this is in place, it becomes a relatively easy decision to make resistance band training part of that overall training routine.

1. QUIT MAKING YOUR BODY 'WALK BACKWARDS'

Our body was designed to walk primarily forward which is why when I watch people exercise on machines it's like they are forcing the body to 'walk backwards'. The body just wasn't designed to exercise on a machine. Maybe that is why most of my physical therapy clients avoided them.

The body is made up of 365 rubber bands called muscles. Each of them needs to be stretched before they can produce force to move the body. Sound familiar?? It should. That is exactly how a rubber band functions. Stretching it makes it explode. So training muscles, using a tool that functions like a muscle, makes a ton of sense.

Now add to that the incredibly quick results you get in improved dynamic flexibility, real world strength, power production along with the elimination of joint pain, and you have a training routine that is going somewhere.

2. DOES YOUR DUMBBELL DO THIS??

Any way you shake it, throw it, or lift it: a weight is a weight and ultimately ….. It only goes where gravity takes it. Not so with resistance bands. Resistance bands defy gravity and allow you to create force horizontally, rotationally, laterally and, like weights, vertically. Just like what happens in life. Maybe that is why when bands become the primary resistance, your body becomes more flexible, gets leaner and learns how to produce force quicker in multiple directions.

3. A BARBELL CANNOT DO THIS??

You can't stretch with a barbell but you can stretch with a resistance band.

Resistance bands are not just for strengthening. Bands are one of the best stretching tools every created. They accommodate and provide a gradual stretch that your muscles prefer. Compare band stretching especially to using some static strap, or having some partner crank on you and the decision becomes very easy to make. Lack of flexibility is one of the top two reasons why injuries occur. It only makes sense that we all better be working on it.

We also know that static, long-hold stretching has been shown not to work and that continuous movement-based stretching with bands is far more effective. I don't know about you, but if I am going to spend my valuable exercise time on flexibility, I prefer it be on something that works.

4. WHERE IS THE GYM LOCATED TODAY??

One of the biggest struggles with sustaining a consistent exercise program is eliminating boredom. One the best ways to eliminate boredom is by training in multiple locations with multiple exercise options that require varying resistance to make the body react and adapt. Yes, you can carry around dumbbells but I find the set-up becomes the workout. Your other option is to carry in a backpack, three to four pairs of resistance bands that provide as much as 300 pounds of resistance and weigh less than five pounds.

It is your decision, but for me, filling up a backpack and taking it anywhere I want to workout is a lot less work and a whole lot more fun!

5. WARNING...ATHLETES ONLY!!

"I can't do that," is what I hear when people come to www. resistancebandtraining.com and watch some of the training videos for the first time. Please understand that bands are being used in all facets of fitness and human performance. I have patients rehabilitating with bands, I have fitness enthusiasts getting great workouts with bands and I have national championship football teams getting super fast training with bands.

Where do you fit in??

Interestingly enough, they all do many of the same basic exercises. It just depends on your strength, power and conditioning levels when it comes to choosing the correct progression.

Bands don't strengthen or improve muscles, they strengthen and improve movements which are driven by muscles. You can never be too good or too strong at moving, regardless if it is on the athletic field or on the field of life.

6. BURNING FAT... BUILDING MUSCLE

FACT...The best way to burn fat is through interval strength training routines. Strength training with bands is different in that you have to work harder where you are weaker and you have to push through the full range of motion. As a result, it will make you work harder, which is what it takes to reach your fat loss goals.

Also, bands make going from exercise to exercise very seamless. Usually all it takes is repositioning your hands or feet and you are set for the next exercise challenge. No changing pins, no adding weights and definitely no sitting around.

As I mentioned earlier, muscles are dumb. They do not think and they definitely do not know what is making them work. All they know is they better get busy reacting and eventually adapting. This means getting more muscle recruited and working. More muscle working means more calories being burnt. This means you stop avoiding mirrors and start getting back the body you like seeing.

The days of resistance band training being the last alternative to building a better body are over. The fitness enthusiast, athlete, coach or fitness professional who has already implemented bands into their program are getting the results that other traditional gym goers, magazine readers or infomercial watchers are still looking for.

"Getting BETTER with BANDS" is not a theory anymore. It's a proven fact that will withstand the test of time and not disappear after eight weeks – like most fitness or performance fads do.

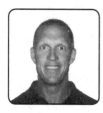

ABOUT DAVID

David Schmitz (aka... The Band Man) is the Co-Owner of Resistance Band Training Systems, LLC and the creator of **www.resistancebandtraining.com,** the only website exclusively devoted to training with large continuously looped resistance bands. Dave's unique professional background and vast experience as an orthopedic physical therapist, performance enhancement specialist, certified strength and conditioning specialist along with his 27 plus years of living fitness and performance training, has allowed him to turn a simple 41 inch resistance band into an incredible multifaceted total training experience for thousands of athletes and fitness enthusiasts around the world, while helping hundreds of fitness professionals and coaches help get their clients or athletes BETTER with BANDS.

What initially started out as a small basement band gym in his home has evolved into an international full service online and offline fitness company. Resistance Band Training Systems, LLC and **www.resistancebandtraining.com** were never created to sell bands. Rather it has always been about teaching and training everyone on why resistance bands were a necessity, not an alternative, when it came to developing training and performance programs that get fast and effective results. Even with a growing online business, Dave continues to run his own adult fitness boot camps and monthly athletic performance camps – while working in the clinic with hundreds of physical therapy patients. He also continues to lecture around the country, teaching coaches and fitness professionals on how to effectively train with resistance bands.

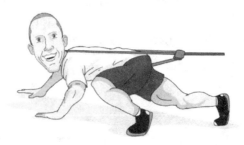

Dave's passion and pursuit of knowledge has allowed him to create over 12 DVDs and write hundreds of articles on the Art of Resistance Band Training and Conditioning. As a result, it is not a surprise or an accident that Dave Schmitz has become nationally known as "The BAND MAN".

To learn more about Resistance Band Training, Dave Schmitz, and 'How to train with Bands', go to **www.resistancebandtraining.com**. You can stay connected with "The BAND MAN" by signing up for Dave's weekly RBT Live Newsletter, joining his Face Book Fan club or by simply following him on Twitter.

CHAPTER 20

FIVE STEP ACTION PLAN TO WIN THE FAT LOSS GAME

BY RYAN KETCHUM

F at loss is a tricky game. Unfortunately most people go about playing this game the wrong way and it ends up costing them a lot. They lose time, their health, their personal enjoyment, and sometimes, their life. There are a lot of ways to approach fat loss and see some success. Our goal is to discover the fastest, safest, and most effective way to lose fat. It isn't easy and it requires a lot of work, but I can promise you that it is all worth it in the end.

How do I know what fat loss is all about? Forget about my degree, certifications, and continuing education. I can honestly tell you that not only am I in the trenches every single day coaching fat loss clients, but I have been on this journey myself. I know the pressures, emotions, and struggles that you go through on a daily basis.

I was never a skinny kid, and I even wore the *husky* size Wrangler jeans growing up. I can't tell you how embarrassing it was to have to wear those around. I was blessed with athletic talent and excelled at sports. I was big and strong, but I was still fat, I just didn't know it at the time. As my educational and athletic career developed, I chose to attend college where I really hit rock bottom. I ballooned to 335 pounds at my heaviest, but never questioned it because I was an NCAA scholarship athlete. I had to be big to perform well in my sport.

I have battled with my weight for as long as I can remember. I tried fat loss pills during the summer when I was 16. I would lift and run. I did all of the things you are supposed to do to lose weight, but I never had consistent success. All through college, every off season from July to October was spent trying to lose weight. I was doing some type of exercise for 2 or 3 hours a day, 4 or 5 days a week. I would try to eat healthy, although I really had no idea what that meant at the time.

I rode the weight loss rollercoaster. Losing 10, 15 or 20 lbs and then gaining it back quicker each time. Frustrated, I told myself that I was a big guy and would never be in great shape. The fact is that I did not know how to get into great shape, not that I could never be in great shape.

As my life changed course, I went from a competitive athlete to personal trainer and business owner. I quickly came to the realization that I needed to make some positive changes in my life. After all, a 300 pound personal trainer isn't the best role model or advertisement. I was finally ready to accept some responsibility and take some serious action. I wanted to regain control over my life.

I began researching fat loss and nutrition tirelessly. I needed to figure out what really worked. I knew that I hated cardio and it didn't really help me before. I knew that counting calories wasn't working for me. So I bought every single informational product and read every bit of fat loss information that I could find to figure out what I needed to do. I literally spent 18 months trying out different programs and seeing the different results. This was the best thing that I ever did. It allowed me to look past the individual programs, diets, and workouts and see the underlying principles that made each of them work. They were all very similar.

18 months and 110 lbs later I was as fit as I had ever been and enjoying every minute of it! Because of this journey and my continued experiences with fat loss, I am able to help hundreds of clients every week get the results they have always dreamed about. I am able to cut through the garbage and give them the principles to a sound fat loss program.

In my journey, both with myself and with my clients, I have come up with a 5-step action plan that must occur to guarantee your success on a fat loss plan.

1. GET THE RIGHT MINDSET

If your head is not 'in the right place', and if you are not ready to make some sacrifices and to take on the challenge, then you might as well not even try. You have to be ready to wage war with your fat loss program. Be ready to overcome adversity from your friends, family, and sometimes even your spouse. If you have the right mindset, you can accomplish anything!

Setting goals for yourself, taking 'before' pictures and choosing someone to hold you accountable, are great first steps to take to ensure success. Set goals that are challenging, yet attainable and reasonable. Know what you want to accomplish, the time frame, and the steps that are needed to meet your goal.

No one wants to take 'before' pictures. They are embarrassing! Rest assured that no one will care what you looked like before if you have made progress and look great now. Use your 'before' pictures as a trophy. They are your bragging rights for getting great results and having success. Your 'before' pictures should be taken from the front in a relaxed stance and from the side. You should take these in a bathing suit or tight and revealing clothing. This will give you the best idea of your current condition.

Many people hire a personal trainer for the accountability factor. Clients will stay with trainers for years, because they know they need to have a scheduled appointment to get in consistent workouts. One of the greatest motivators for success is feeling like you cannot let someone down. Finding a friend or family member that you can confide in and keep updated on your progress, will greatly increase the chances for your success. Openly talking about your goals and your quest will make you think twice about cheating on your dinner, or skipping your workout.

2. SET ASIDE SMALL BLOCKS OF TIME TO DEVOTE ENTIRELY TOWARDS FAT LOSS

I like to tackle fat loss in 4-8 week blocks with my clients. If they are beginners, we will gradually get them started on our training programs and nutrition so that they see results. Once we have established this foundation we will aggressively attack their fat loss goals with a focused program for 4-8 week blocks.

After this block we will bring them back to a maintenance phase for 1-2 weeks to let them recover mentally, emotionally and physically. Then we attack again until we hit their goals. The 1-2 week recovery period is not a free for all! It is also a directed and focused program that is healthy, but not as aggressive as the larger blocks. Often times we still see dramatic fat loss in this phase.

Mentally, it is easier to have a start and end point for your aggressive fat loss plan. Most people can commit to a program for a few weeks and see great results. *Having a long-term plan is important, but knowing that you can break it down into short bursts towards your goal makes it more achievable.*

This has many benefits mentally but also physiologically. It gives the body a chance to rest and reset its level of homeostasis at a new weight. Many experts will tell you that the body will find a set point at which it feels comfortable. When your body finds this set point, it will fight to stay within a comfortable range. The bursts of aggressive fat loss followed by brief maintenance phases allow the body to find a new set point but not get comfortable for long.

3. PLAN AND PREPARE

What are you going to eat and when? What happens if you get caught up at work or on the road and you can't eat what you are supposed to? Do you have a backup plan? What is your training program going to consist of? The more you know and the more obstacles that you can identify early in the process, the better equipped you will be to handle them.

4. FOLLOW A SOUND NUTRITION PROGRAM

A fat loss program is incomplete if you are not following a sound nutritional plan. You will never see great success without making sure you are fueling your body for fat loss. There are many different concepts, diets, and plans that will work. The key is finding the one that works for you and being consistent. Pick a plan that will fit your lifestyle, goal, and personality. If you are great at sticking to a plan and following instructions, then a plan that lays out all of your meals for you over the course of month is a great idea. However, if you need some flexibility you might want a plan that allows some freedom with your food choices, but follows sound principles for fat loss.

5. IMPLEMENT AN EFFECTIVE FAT LOSS TRAINING PROGRAM

The fat loss program you choose should include tissue quality, mobility, core, strength and metabolic work. A program should also take into consideration your current fitness level, previous training history, injuries, and availability. *Safe, effective,* and *brief* are three words that come to mind when picking a fat loss program.

One of the biggest problems with fat loss programs, right along with ineffective nutrition plans, is ineffective, outdated training programs. The days of 'hours on the treadmill' and doing 'boring body-part' split workouts are long gone. Real world results are showing us that 45 minute or less workouts, full body routines and metabolic conditioning, are the most effective way to drop fat.

Here is what a training day should look like:

> 5 minutes of foam rolling and tissue quality work such as tennis ball massage, stick massage, etc.
> 10 minutes of dynamic warm up and movement prep
> 20-25 minutes Strength work (including core)
> 10-15 minutes of metabolic conditioning work
> 5 minutes of stretching or tissue quality work

This is 50-55 minutes of total time in the gym. Only 40 minutes of that is high intensity work.

You only need to perform workouts such as this three times per week for great results. If you are short on time each day, you can certainly split up the time spent in the gym. You can separate the strength and metabolic work on alternate days, performing one day with 20 minutes of dedicated strength work and the next day with 20 minutes of metabolic work.

We need to include two or three segments of training in our program to get great results. These segments are strength work, metabolic conditioning, and active recovery. There is also a period of rest that should be taken weekly.

Here is what a weekly schedule might look like for a person training just three days a week for optimal results:

Monday: Strength and Metabolic
Tuesday: Active Recovery
Wednesday: Strength and Metabolic
Thursday: Active Recovery
Friday: Strength and Metabolic
Saturday: Active Recovery
Sunday: Rest

If you wanted to train for a shorter period of time on 5-6 days per week we would need the schedule to look like this:

Monday: Strength
Tuesday: Metabolic
Wednesday: Strength
Thursday: Metabolic
Friday: Strength
Saturday: Metabolic or Active Recovery
Sunday: Rest

Note: Strength work is designated as resistance training.

A strength program might look something like this:

1A Plank 3 x 30s
1B Cable Wood Chop 3 x 15 each side
Rest 30s

2A DB Squat 3 x 12
2B Chin Up 3 x 12
Rest 30s
3A Reverse Lunge 3 x 12 each side
3B Push Up 3 x 12
Rest 30s

In this workout the exercises are labeled with a number and letter. The number is the group of exercises and the order in which they are to be performed. The letter is the order within the group. For example, in groups 1A and 1B we would perform the plank for 30 seconds and immediately go into the cable wood chop for 15 repetitions on each side followed by a 30 second rest. We would then complete this 2 more times for a total of 3 sets each before moving on to the next exercise pairing.

This will keep you moving at a good pace and get in a great full body workout.

Metabolic conditioning workouts are set up to increase the heart rate, increase the respiratory rate, and cause the body to burn calories at a higher rate over an extended period of time. Body weight, kettlebell, medicine ball, band, and calisthenics movements are great for this type of conditioning.

Here is what a metabolic session might look like:

1A KB Swing 40 seconds
Rest 20 seconds
1B Push Up 40 seconds
Rest 20 seconds
1C Squat Thrust 40 seconds
Rest 20 seconds
1D Medicine Ball Slams 40 seconds.
Rest 20 seconds

You would complete 5 rounds total if you did this as a stand-alone workout or complete 2-3 rounds if you did this at the end of a strength workout.

Active recovery days are placed in the weekly schedule to keep you motivated and help you enjoy fitness. These days should be spent doing some type of activity that you truly enjoy doing. This could be walking the dog, playing with your kids, shooting hoops, walking a round of golf, or any other of the thousands of activities that bring you pleasure. The idea is to stay active but allow your body time to heal.

If you are ready to change your life forever and increase your chances of success, you need to be taking these 5 actions and implementing them today. Get your mindset in order, set your goals, prepare and plan for success, find your nutrition program and implement the fat loss training program. It really is that simple. Start your fat loss journey on the right foot and set yourself up for success.

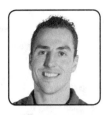

ABOUT RYAN

Ryan Ketchum is co-owner of Force Fitness and Performance in Bloomington, Indiana. He has helped hundreds of clients lose unwanted fat and regain control over their lives. Ryan is known for his effective fat loss training systems that incorporate goal setting, training programs and sound nutrition to get results fast.

Ryan's expertise in the field of weight loss and fitness came about from using his years of training as an athlete and the incredible knowledge he gained from his own experiences, combined with his education as a kinesiology student at Indiana University, to transform his own body from 330 lbs to 220 lbs in just a year's time.

This incredible transformation that Ryan undertook, required tremendous will power and self-confidence, both qualities that he instills in all his clients.

WWW.BEFORCEFIT.COM

CHAPTER 21

THE LAST MINUTE BEACH BODY:

A BLUE PRINT FOR BUSY PEOPLE LOOKING TO DROP BODY FAT, LOSE INCHES AND TONE UP IN ONLY 14 DAYS

BY JOE CARABASE, CPT AND IYCA NUTRITION SPECIALIST

Do you not have enough time? Studies show us that people's top excuse for not exercising is *lack of time.* We all share a common goal: *to look better naked.* Although the specifics of the goal will differ from person to person, I have never met anybody nor do I think anyone exists who does not want to look better naked.

We all have good intentions on hitting this goal yet we all blame there not being enough time. There's work, family, friends, social events, change of the season, blah, blah, blah, and not enough time to go around. Although people are not happy with their situations, they are willing to accept it until one of three things happens:

1. New Years: As cliché as it is, social pressure forces us to rethink

our approach to fitness every January

2. Vacation: Whether married or single, no one wants to look nor feel like the fat person when they vacation
3. Summer: Beaches, BBQ's and warm weather make it hard to hide under sweaters and suits.

When any of the aforementioned events arises, we try to reverse bad habits and the inactive lifestyle in *last chance* efforts to change the way we look and feel. Yet, unless you are genetically gifted or could afford the right fitness professional help, chances are you were never able to accomplish your goals.

Until now. *The Last Minute Beach Body* program is designed for the sole purpose of dropping body fat and toning up in two weeks.

Why two weeks? Is that even enough time?

Through extensive trial and error, I have found two weeks to be the shortest amount of time you can make serious change. Due to the level of commitment and intensity of the *Last Minute Beach Body,* your body will respond by dropping body fat, inches off your waist and increased muscle definition.

Is the *Last Minute Beach Body* something you can maintain?

No. In fact it would be unhealthy to maintain longer than two weeks. This high intensity program is specifically designed to get your mind and body right in a boot camp style two week period.

Who is this program created for?

Everyone. Allergies aside, the nutritional segment of this program will help anyone shed unwanted fat. The fitness segment offers various levels of difficulty so whether you are new to working out or been getting after it for a while, your body will be forced to respond.

NUTRITIONAL SECTION

BREAKING BAD HABITS

You don't have to do it all at once or cut out all sugars. If you currently find yourself with any sort of sugar addiction, I recommend you start by getting rid of the least measureable high sugar foods in your diet (fast foods, processed/refined foods, sodas and fruit drinks) before committing to this program. This process should not take longer than 10 days. If you find yourself experiencing symptoms of withdrawal, from these foods, reduce your sugar and caffeine more gradually. To assist in this process, replace your craving with a piece of fruit or ONE small piece of dark chocolate. It is not recommended to go from 0 (high sugar-processed food diet) to 60 (Last Minute Beach Body program) overnight.

THE FOUNDATION

The meals in this diet are structured via my carb timing approach, which will make sure your body uses these calories as energy and not store them as fat. The typical American diet gives us more carbohydrates then we need.

By eliminating most traditional carbohydrates and wheat products from your diet, you will by default take in less overall calories. Moreover, wheat products often cause you to bloat and store calories around your midsection.

Aside from blueberries, fruit is left out of this plan as the sugars will slow down your fat burning process.

DO THESE DAILY

1. Eat Breakfast: Not being hungry or again, not having enough time are not going to cut it here! Breakfast is vital to reach your optimal performance both physically and mentally. Moreover, "breaking the fast," will give your body the necessary fuel to keep your metabolism running and storing calories.
2. Drink 0.55 x your body weight in ozs. of water. This formula will give you the right amount of water that will help your body function properly and keep you hydrated and full. I recommend buying a 32 oz, BPA free sustainable water bottle and carrying it with you throughout the day.
3. Eat four small meals: Although this program is restrictive, I hate requiring clients measure everything they eat especially since you are required to eat so much. IF you have a hard time eating four meals, reduce the serving sizes. This however should not

be an issue, if you are keeping up with the workouts, your body will need the fuel! If you're still hungry, add more greens!

4. 'Graze' in between meals and before bed: Snacking tends to give people the wrong idea. People associate snacking with empty calories and inevitable body fat. In reality, *snacking* or *grazing* will keep your metabolism working all day, providing you with energy and helping your body burn calories.

5. Eat after dinner and before bed: Your body needs these calories in order to build muscle and burn calories overnight!

6. Prepare: Set aside 30 minutes before bed to get your food ready for tomorrow. Pack all meals in Tupperware along with ice in a cooler/lunch box. Yes I know, a bit extreme, but you want to shed body fat in two weeks, right?

7. Ignore the negative: There will be people questioning what you're doing, just forgive them for their insecurities. Focus on the end result, a more slim, happier and confident you.

8. Make sure to schedule a workout 60 – 90 minutes after a meal.

WHAT DO I DO IF...?

1. I go out to eat:
   a. Politely share with your party what you are setting off to accomplish, this will prevent you from feeling guilty and/or peer pressure
   b. Drink 16-32 ozs of water one hour before you arrive
   c, Scale the menu before arriving to find a way to eat as close to this plan as possible
   d. Have a salad as an appetizer
   e. Ask for what you want and don't feel guilty: The restaurant's role is to serve you. Asking for oil and vinegar, no bread, vegetable substitutes, no butter etc.. are necessary for you to achieve a more lean body

2. If you are not full or not satisfied you can:
   a. Eat unlimited greens and beans
   b. Only in extreme cravings, allow yourself one piece of dark chocolate or one piece of fruit. Go into a quiet room and slowly eat whatever it is (PROPORTIONED!) – enjoy every second of it.

THE PLAN

Breakfast: No later than 30 minutes after you wake up	1. 2:1 egg white to egg ratio with spinach and tomatoes 2. Breakfast shake: ¾ cup of oatmeal, one scoop of Prograde Protein, a table spoon of olive oil (or flax seeds) , ¼ cup of blueberries and ½ water ½ Organic Lactose and Fat Free milk
Grazing options: Aim for one in between each meal. If you need more flavor for the veggies, drizzle vinegar over them	1. One handful of carrots, diced bell peppers, broccoli 2. One handful of raw almonds or walnuts
After dinner and before bed: One serving – NO fruit!	1. One serving plain Greek yogurt 2. One serving of 1% cottage cheese 3. One cup of Organic Lactose and Fat Free milk
Post workout: Consume within 30 minutes	1. One – two scoops of Prograde Protein. If you're new to weight training and protein, take one scoop, otherwise two. Mixed with a ¼ of blueberries and Organic Lactose and Fat Free milk
Lunch and dinner: Pick and choose one from each category	I. 4-6 oz Lean grass fed organic meat, 4-6 oz lean organic chicken, 4:2 egg whites to egg, or 4-6 oz of white fish or salmon II. 1-2 cups of organic spinach or organic mixed greens or, asparagus, diced bell peppers, broccoli III. ¼ -1/2 cup of kidney, garbanzo or black beans IV. Lemon, lime, hot sauce, olive oil (applied after) or vinegar

---

GROCERY LIST: The most effective way for you to grocery shop is to bring this list and only buy what's on this list

1. Organic eggs
2. Lean grass fed organic meat, lean organic chicken, white fish or salmon
3. Organic Lactose and Fat Free milk
4. Plain Greek yogurt
5. 1% cottage cheese
6. Dry oats
7. Organic spinach or mixed greens
8. Kidney, black and/or garbanzo beans
9. Prograde Protein
10. Frozen blueberries
11. Lemon or lime
12. Extra virgin olive oil
13. Vinegar
14. Hot sauce (optional)

FITNESS SECTION

The 12 Components:

1. Elevated Activity: To ensure the caloric burning potential, you need to increase your amount of movement in everyday life: walk when possible rather then drive, park farther away, take the stairs, replace your office chair with a stability ball – wherever you have the opportunity to be more functional!

2. Interval workouts: Rather than working out for an hour straight, you will have *interval workouts* broken down to as much as 45 minutes straight and as little as 4 minutes straight at different times throughout the day. This allows for your body to maximize intensity in each session by providing rest in between.

3. All out Intensity: The workouts in this program are designed to be performed at YOUR maximum effort, priming your body for the most effective fat burning and hormonal benefits. This doesn't mean you have to work out until you faint (listen to your body) or that you should be grunting during each rep (although

you could…)

4. Multi-joint movements: The purpose of these exercises is to tax your body by using multiple muscles at once.

5. Cardio strength training: During resistance training, your heart rate should be cranked up, allowing you to get cardio in addition to your strength training.

6. Light walk and Yoga movements on days 8 and 14 will stretch your muscles and lower blood cortisol levels.

7. Warm-up before exercising: This will get your core temperature up, distribute blood to working muscles and preparing your body to work. Perform the warm-up below before all training routines.

8. Cool-down after exercising: Move around at a slow pace to bring your heart rate down for five – 10 minutes. Precede this with a full body stretch.

9. Self Myofascial release (optional): SMR with a foam roll will reduce adhesion and scar tissue accumulation.

10. Timed set: Each routine is designed using a work:rest ratio. This means you work for a period of time and rest for a period of time, e.g., 50:10, work for 50 seconds, rest 10 seconds. Workout sequences allow for each individual to do the most quality reps that individual can perform.

11. The amount of sets is left open, therefore you are performing the amount of sets your current fitness level can handle.
    - Beginner: Less then six months of consistent resistance training should perform 1-3 sets
    - Novice: Consistent resistance training for 6-12 months should perform 2-4 sets.
    - Advanced: Consistent resistance training for over a year should perform 3-6 sets.

12. For both cardio strength-training routines, there are three levels for each exercise. You are only to perform ONE level per set. The following are recommendations, based on the categories above:
    - Beginner: Level 1 and 2
    - Novice: Level 2 and 3
    - Advanced: Level 3

THE PLAN

Scheduled Workouts	Workout sequence	Sets
Day 1: Cardio Strength Training Routine A	50:10	1-5
Day 2: Bodyweight Training Routine A	30:10	1-5
Day 3: Interval Training A	n/a	12
Day 4: Cardio Strength Training Routine B	50:10	1-5
Day 5: Interval Training B	n/a	10
Day 6: Cardio Strength Training Routine A	50:10	1-5
Day 7: Yoga Training	30:10	3-5
Day 8: Cardio Strength Training Routine B	40:20	2-6
Day 9: Bodyweight Training Routine B	40:10	2-6
Day 3: Interval Training A and C	n/a	12 and 4-8
Day 4: Cardio Strength Training Routine A	40:20	3-7
Day 5: Interval Training B and D	n/a	10 and 8
Day 6: Cardio Strength Training Routine B	40:10	3-7
Day 7: Yoga Training B	30:10	4-6

THE WARM-UP

Directions: Perform the following exercises back to back, rest 30 seconds and repeat two more times	
Spiderman Lunge	5 reps each side
High Knee Pull	5 reps each side
Y – W	10 reps
Crouch to Straight Leg	10 reps

BODYWEIGHT TRAINING ROUTINES

BODYWEIGHT TRAINING ROUTINE A

Directions: Perform exercises 1-5 back to back, rest 45 seconds and repeat. After you complete the appropriate amount of sets, complete the Finisher.

1.   Level I: Wall Push-up
     Level II: Isometric Push-up
     Level III: Isometric Negative Push-up

2.	Level I: Split Squat with T hold Level II: Split Squat with Y hold Level III: Split Squat with I hold* For the following exercises, hold the end position for three seconds before returning
3.	Level I: Renegade Row against wall Level II: Renegade Row on knees Level III: Renegade Row*
4.	Level I: 45 degree Wall sit with T hold Level II: Wall Sit with T hold Level III: Single Leg Wall Sit
5.	Level I: Plank against wall Level II: Plank Level III: Plank with arm Pull in
The Finisher: 28 squats 14 squat jumps 14 lateral lunges 28 lateral jumps Rest 60 seconds and repeat	

*To increase difficulty, add weight or an additional 10 seconds

BODYWEIGHT TRAINING ROUTINE B

Directions: Perform exercises 1-5 back to back, rest 45 seconds and repeat. After you complete the appropriate amount of sets, complete the Finisher.	
1.	Level I: Wall Push-up Level II: Push-up Level III: Vertical Push-up
2.	Level I: Lateral Lunge with a T hold Level II: Lateral lunge with a Y Raise Level III: 180 degree lunge
3.	Level I: Y to W Level II: Y to W Squat Level III: Y to W Squat Jump

4.	Level I: Side plank on hips Level II: Side plank Level III: Side plank with scapula rotation
5.	Level I: Stand to push-up Level II: Squat Thrust Level III: Squat thrust with jump
	The Finisher: 20 Push-ups (the most advanced progression you can perform 20 push-ups without a rest) 10 squat thrusts 10 mountain climbers (right leg – left leg = 1 rep) 20 Squat thrusts with jump Rest 60 seconds and repeat

*To increase difficulty, add weight or an additional 10 seconds

CARDIO STRENGTH TRAINING ROUTINES

CARDIO STRENGTH TRAINING ROUTINE A

Directions: Perform exercises 1-3 back to back, rest 20 seconds then perform exercises 4 & 5. Rest 20 seconds and repeat the appropriate amount of sets then complete the Finisher.	
1.	Level I: Kettlebell Swings Level II: Kettlebell Swing with two kettlebells Level III Alternate Kettle Bell Swings
2.	Level I: Front Squat Level II: Partial Squat to Press Level III: Squat to Press
3.	Level I: Walk out Level II: Walk out to push-up Level III: Walk out to vertical push-up
4.	Level I: Reverse Lunge Level II: Reverse lunge with a raise Level III: Bulgarian squat with a raise
5.	Inverted Row*

> **The Finisher:** Perform five explosive reps of the Kettlebell swings and walk outs, rest five seconds starting after you walk back up and grab the kettlebell and repeat. Repeat for three sets.

*Start off with your chest more vertical, to progress, walk your feet out to increase the range of motion. (*Ref. pg.196)

CARDIO STRENGTH TRAINING ROUTINE B

Directions: Perform 1-3 back to back, rest 20 seconds then perform exercises 4 &5. Rest 20 seconds and repeat the appropriate amount of sets then complete the Finisher.
1. Level I: Romanian deadlift Level II Romanian deadlift with biceps curl Level III: Romanian deadlift with biceps curl to overhead press
2. Kettle bell or Dumbbell High Pull*
3. Level I: Assisted Pull-ups Level II: Pull-ups Level III: Side to side pull ups
4. Level : Lunge Level II: Lunge with frontal rotation Level III: Lunge with overhead rotation
5. Level I: Step-up Level II: Step-up holding dumbbells Level III: Step-up with biceps curl
The Finisher: High Pull Tabata: Perform as many reps of the high pull as possible in 20 seconds, rest 10 seconds and repeat seven times

Start off with no weight to learn form, once you feel comfortable, progress this movement by increasing the intensity of each rep and adding higher weight. (Ref. #2 above)

CARDIO WORKOUTS

A. STATIONARY BIKE INTERVAL TRAINING ROUTINE

Movements	Work Level	Work Duration	Intensity	Rest level	Rest Duration	Number of intervals
Slow jog/run	6	3-5 minutes	5/10	n/a	n/a	
Sprint	9	30 seconds	9/10	5	15 seconds	12
Cool down walk/jog	3	3-10 minutes	3/10	n/a	n/a	1

B. OUTDOOR INTERVAL TRAINING ROUTINE

Movements	Distance	Intensity	Rest	Number of intervals
Heel To Butt, Lateral Lunge Forward High Knee Skip	20 yards each	5/10	Perform each movement back to back	2 each movement
Sprint	100 yards	9/10	Light jog back to starting point	10
Cool down walk/jog	100 yards down and back	3/10	n/a	1

C. PERFORM THE FOLLOWING MOVEMENTS IN SEQUENCE, RESTING 45 SECONDS AFTER MOUNTAIN CLIMBERS

Movements	Work Level	Work Duration	Intensity	Rest level	Rest Duration	Number of Sets
Jumping jacks	9	50 reps	9/10	n/a	n/a	4-8
Squat Jumps	9	10 reps	9/10	n/a	n/a	4-8
Squat Thrusts	9	10 reps	3/10	n/a	n/a	4-8
Mountain Climbers	9	30 seconds	9/10	3/10	45 seconds	4-8

D. ELLIPTICAL OR TREADMILL INTERVAL TRAINING ROUTINE

Movements	Work Level	Work Duration	Intensity	Rest level	Rest Duration	Number of intervals
Slow jog/run	6	3-5 minutes	5/10	n/a	n/a	1
Sprint	9	60 seconds	9/10	5	30 seconds	8
Cool down walk/jog	3	3-10 minutes	3/10	n/a	n/a	

YOGA ROUTINE

Directions: Walk for 30 minutes then complete the following poses, back to back for the appropriate amount of sets.

Poses	Duration	Sets
Downward Facing Dog Pose	30 seconds	3
Standing Forward Bend	30 seconds	3
Triangle Pose	30 seconds	3
Warrior Pose	30 seconds	3
Extended Side Angle Pose	30 seconds	3

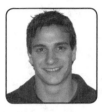

ABOUT JOE

Joe Carabase, also known as "The Results Coach," is a fitness expert that has not only helped hundreds of people lose thousands of pounds of fat, but has also inspired people to develop healthy lifestyles and changed their lives. Joe has been seen on NBC and Fox affiliates. Joe founded his company, LBN Fitness, LLC in 2008 to provide people with a simplistic approach to look and feel better naked. Since then, Joe has built an online following through his informative yet entertaining blog, www.carabasetraining.com.

"The Results Coach" also is the owner of M.E.L.T Fitness Studio in Connecticut where Joe and his team of trainers coach people of all fitness levels to transform their mind and bodies through their unique style of semi-private training and bootcamps. In addition to his on and offline fitness businesses, Joe is the director of a Professional Fitness Program at Branford Hall Career Institute in Connecticut.

To learn more about Joe Carabase and to receive the free Special Report "21 Ways to Look Better Naked," visit www.carabasetraining.com.

www.carabasetraining.com

www.thelastminutebeachbody.com

www.meltfitnesstudio.com

CHAPTER 22

BUILDING A BETTER MEAL PLAN

BY JAYSON HUNTER AND JIM LABADIE

There are many ways to build a meal plan. The most common one and also the most frustrating is the calorie-counting method. It seems great because you will know exactly every calorie you consume, but you also easily get frustrated trying to track every calorie when you really don't have to.

CONVERTING CALORIES TO FOOD EXCHANGES

There's another way to plan your meals besides counting calories – with something called food exchanges. Why convert calories to exchanges? Because your life is too busy to count calories all day long. Tallying up calories is not an efficient way to eat healthfully day-in and day-out. Plus, it's time-consuming and a bit neurotic to track every last calorie you eat.

Look, in the grand scheme of eating well, it doesn't matter if an apple amounts to 68 calories or 74 calories. Does it? What counts is the healthy choices you make each day. Many people lose weight without ever counting a single calorie.

So why did I have you calculate that formula for your daily caloric needs? I want you to have a baseline of calories, so you can determine your food exchanges.

WHAT ARE FOOD EXCHANGES?

A "food exchange" is a fancy way of describing something you're already familiar with: serving sizes! Here's how it works: As you may know, there are 6 main food categories.

1. Dairy
2. Vegetable
3. Fruit
4. Starch
5. Protein
6. Fat

Each of these categories has a calorie guideline that equals **1 serving of food** for that category. Some categories also have subcategories (such as with Dairy and Protein below). For example:

Dairy:

Low fat: 1 serving = 90 calories
Reduced fat: 1 serving = 120 calories
Whole-milk products: 1 serving = 150 calories

Vegetable: 1 serving = 25 calories

Fruit: 1 serving = 60 calories

Starch: (bread, cereal, rice, pastas): 1 serving = 80 calories

Protein:

Lean protein and meat substitutes (0 to 3 grams of fat): 1 serving = 35 to 55 calories, respectively
Medium-fat protein and meat substitutes: 1 serving = 75 calories
High-fat protein and meat substitutes: 1 serving = 100 calories

Fat: 1 serving = 45 calories

Appendix A in this book explains what foods equal 1 serving for each of the above groups. The information there is designed to help you meet your daily serving requirements with foods you enjoy. For example, 1 oz. of plain chicken breast equals 1 serving of protein. But you may choose a 2-oz. chicken breast flavored with low-calorie marinade. That equals 2 servings of protein. You will also be able to dine at a restaurant or friend's place and still determine how many calories are on your plate.

HOW TO CONVERT CALORIES TO FOOD EXCHANGES

Now it's time to convert your calorie needs to exchanges. I will explain how to do this manually, but you can also refer to the exchange lists for different calorie counts in Appendix B.

To manually convert calories to servings sizes, determine your proper nutrient ratio. So, if you've reached your weight loss goals and want to maintain your new, thin body, your nutrient ratio should be around 45% carbohydrates, 35% protein and 20% fat.

For example, let's say your calorie needs are 1,450 calories per day. You would do the following calculations:

1,450 x 45% (carbs) = 652 calories
1,450 x 35% (protein) = 507 calories
1,450 x 20% (fat) = 290 calories

These are the calories you need to eat from each nutrient ratio.

Carbohydrates: 652 calories
Protein: 507 calories
Fat: 290 calories

Now it gets a bit trickier because you have to know how many grams of these nutrients are in each exchange category. Don't worry, I'm not going to give you more formulas to work out. Simply go to Appendix B and find the allotted number of calories you should be eating in a day (e.g., 1,800, 2,000, 2,200, etc.). The numbers in Appendix B are in 100-calorie increments. Round up if your calorie level falls above the halfway mark (e.g., 2,060 = 2,100); round down for calorie levels below the halfway mark (e.g., 2, 040 = 2,000).

An example of how the chart in Appendix B works.

Calories: 1,450 (round up to 1,500)

Ratio: 45/35/20
Dairy: 3
Vegetable: 6
Fruit: 3
Starch: 4
Protein: 11
Fat: 1

TIP: If you exercise 4 to 5 times per week, you need higher carbs. If you're less active or not active at all, you need lower carbs. Modify the exchanges to fit your lifestyle (and work toward creating an active lifestyle for yourself).

LAYING OUT YOUR EXCHANGES

Laying out the 45/35/20 ratio of exchanges is already done for you. Just go to Appendix B and follow the suggested layout of how you should eat throughout the day.

Notice the exchanges are spread out so you eat some type of protein and vegetable at every meal whenever possible. This accomplishes 2 things: 1) you get a variety of nutrients throughout the day, and 2) you efficiently fuel your body to maximize your metabolism.

You don't have to follow the layout in Appendix B exactly. You can create your own plan however you'd like. Just remember to spread your exchanges out as evenly as possible throughout the day.

HOW TO BUILD YOUR MEALS

Remember when your parents doled out the proper portions of food on your plate, then told you to finish everything? This practice was fine when dinner plates were smaller and the entire surface wasn't covered with food.

Dinner plates today are often much larger than they used to be – yet we still fill the entire plate with food! One key way you can maintain a healthy weight is by controlling portion sizes.

Research has shown that people often underestimate how many daily calories they consume by as much as 25%. Until now, I've been explaining a lot about the right kinds of foods to eat for weight loss and maintenance. However, eating the right *amount* of food at each meal is just as important.

Proper portion sizes might be smaller than you realize. Estimating portion size is easy once you know what a proper portion size looks like. Use the portion chart shown below to help give you an idea of typical serving sizes.

Cheese – 1 ounce/28 grams of cheese = 4 dice
Fruit – 1 fruit serving = baseball
Vegetables – ½ cup/120 ml = ½ a baseball
Pasta/rice – ½ cup/120 ml = ½ a baseball
Fish/meat – 1 serving of cooked meat, fish or poultry = deck of cards
Peanut butter – 2 tablespoons/30 ml of peanut butter = large marshmallow
Dairy – 1 cup/240 ml of milk, yogurt = a fist
Butter – 1 teaspoon/5 ml = pat of butter
Bread – 1 serving of carbohydrate = 1 slice
Salad dressing – 2 tablespoons/30 ml = standard ice cube
Potato – ½ a potato = ½ a baseball

When you make your plate for each meal, choose, for example, 1 protein serving, 1 starch/carbohydrate serving and 2 servings of vegetables and/ or a fruit. Using a portion control chart like the one above shows you there should be plenty of empty space on your plate! Overloading your plate leads to overeating.

To properly build a meal, write down your total daily servings, including how many of those servings you should have at each meal. Record the results on a piece of paper or Excel spreadsheet. Now go to Appendix A and choose foods of the appropriate serving sizes. Create your meal plans for multiple days in advance to help keep you compliant with your new approach to eating.

TIP: You can combine servings at one meal. For example, if dinner calls for 5 oz. of protein, you can have a 5 oz. chicken breast instead of breaking it up into 5 separate servings of protein.

FOODS TO SELECT MOST OFTEN

Below is a list of foods that I consider staples in any meal plan. They're nutrient-dense, good for your metabolism and make you feel full. Try to incorporate a variety of these foods into your daily meals.

LEAN PROTEIN SOURCES:

- Chicken or turkey (white meat)
- Tuna fish (canned, in water)
- Lean beef
- Egg whites
- Non-fat cottage cheese
- Fish like shark, salmon, flounder (farmed often have the least contaminants)
- Shellfish

"MEDIUM-FAT" PROTEIN SOURCES:

- Chicken or turkey (dark meat)
- Whole eggs
- Cottage cheese (2% or whole)
- Steaks (moderate-fat cuts, 20 to 25% fat)
- Other meats (moderate fat, 20 to 25% fat)
- Mozzarella cheese (nonfat or skim)

VEGETABLES:

- Broccoli
- Salad (lettuce, romaine lettuce, etc.); use nonfat salad dressing
- Cabbage
- Green beans
- Spinach
- Zucchini
- Squash
- Red or green pepper
- Asparagus
- Carrots
- Tomatoes
- Cauliflower
- Mushrooms
- Artichoke hearts

CARBOHYDRATES:

- Sweet potatoes or yams
- Brown rice
- Corn
- Peas
- Legumes (chickpeas, lima beans, lentils, dry beans)
- High-fiber cereals (All Bran, Fiber One, Grape Nuts, Cracklin' Oat Bran, Shredded Wheat)
- Oats and oatmeal (not instant oatmeal)
- Black beans
- 100% Wholegrain pasta (Eden, Hodgson Mill, Purity Foods)
- 100% Wholegrain bread (Pepperidge Farm, Nature's Path, Nature's Own, Earth Grains)

HIGH-FIBER FRUITS:

- Raspberries
- Strawberries
- Blackberries
- Apples
- Pears
- Prunes
- Oranges

Eating Out: Is It Possible?

What choices do you make when you eat at a restaurant? Can you ever eat out again?

Yes, you can eat out. Many restaurants now have lean or low-calorie meals to accommodate healthy eaters like you. Choose a dish from the restaurant's low-calorie menu, and follow my guidelines for dining out:

- Find fast-food restaurants that grill their meats rather than fry them.
- Choose grilled chicken over a double-patty melt.
- Keep sandwiches plain. Add your own condiments like mustard. Steer clear of a restaurant's special sauces and cheeses.
- Choose a baked potato or beans instead of fries and coleslaw.
- Fill your plate with plenty of vegetables.
- Order salad with dressing on the side; pick oil-and-vinegar

dressings to boost your intake of Omega 3 fatty acids.
- Drink water (not soda) to satisfy thirst and reduce calories.

7 SPECIFIC SUPERFOODS TO INCLUDE IN YOUR DIET EVERY DAY

I have a list of superfoods that I like to include in every client's meal plan. These foods are very nutrient-dense and contain many disease-fighting properties. Here, I share my favorite superfoods with you. Please make them part of your own meal plan.

1. FRUIT

The following fruits are high in antioxidants to help prevent disease. They also contain flavonoids that help with eyesight and coordination. The dark-colored fruits also provide fiber and boost your immune system.

Fruits I especially recommend:

- Raspberries
- Blueberries
- Blackberries
- Guava (great source of lycopene)
- Goji berries
- Dried plums

2. NUTS

Nuts are a great source of fiber, vitamin B6, niacin, magnesium, healthy monounsaturated fats, protein and more. Nuts help lower LDL (bad) cholesterol and may help maintain healthy blood vessels, as well.

Nuts I especially recommend:

- Almonds
- Walnuts
- Cashews
- Brazil nuts
- Hazelnuts

3. BEANS/LENTILS

Beans are a great source of protein and fiber – and they're low in calories. Beans help stabilize blood sugars and provide isoflavones, which help prevent certain forms of cancers and heart disease.

Beans I especially recommend:

- Legumes (chickpeas, lima beans, lentils, dry beans)
- Black beans
- Red beans

4. OILS

Oils – particularly Extra Virgin Olive Oil – are examples of heart-healthy fat that helps lower LDL (bad) cholesterol. Oils contain antioxidant and anti-inflammatory properties, as well. And they help control food cravings.

Oils I especially recommend:

- Extra Virgin Olive Oil
- Fish oil

5. FISH

Fish contains the potent Omega 3 fatty acid, which helps your body store less fat and convert fat to energy. Fish is a great anti-inflammatory and a wonderful "brain food." The ADA recommends 1.5 to 3 grams of Omega 3 fat a day. One serving of the choices below provides almost 4 grams of Omega 3 fat.

Fish I especially recommend:

- Salmon
- Tuna
- Mackerel

6. VEGETABLES

A variety of color is key when selecting vegetables. For example, orange carrots are a great source of beta-carotene, which can reduce the risk of cancer. Red tomatoes contain lycopene, another powerful antioxidant for reducing the risk of cancer. Dark green, leafy vegetables, such as spinach, contain carotenoids that improve your immune system and are full of vitamins and minerals. Broccoli, cauliflower, kale and other cruciferous vegetables contain cancer-fighting properties.

Vegetables I especially recommend:

- Carrots
- Tomatoes
- Broccoli
- Kale
- Spinach
- Cauliflower
- Beets
- Cabbage
- Swiss chard
- Purslane (used as a salad green or herb)

7. GREEN TEA

Not only is non-caffeinated fluid good for you, research shows that green tea may be one of the best disease-fighting beverages you can consume. It's very high in antioxidants and has cancer-fighting properties. Green tea may actually inhibit the growth of cancer cells, according to research. Other research shows it reduces overall cholesterol levels and increases the ratio of HDL (good) cholesterol to LDL (bad) cholesterol.

Here are just some of the ailments that drinking green tea helps:

- cancer
- rheumatoid arthritis
- high cholesterol levels
- cardiovascular disease
- infection
- impaired immune function

Finally, research suggests that drinking green tea also benefits those who want to lose weight. Subjects who consumed caffeine plus green tea extract burned more calories than those who consumed caffeine or a placebo. More studies are needed to determine if this evidence is valid, but so far it looks encouraging.

ABOUT JAYSON

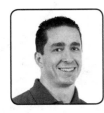

Jayson Hunter RD, CSCS is the author of the Carb Rotation Diet as well as the Director of Research and Development for Prograde Nutrition. He is also a best selling author and contributor for the book: *Big Ideas for Your Business.*

He has also been featured on CBS, ABC, FOX and NBC to discuss his very successful Carb Rotation Diet program.

His nutritional programs have helped thousands of clients successfully lose weight and create permanent lifestyle changes. Jayson's method of eating and nutritional programming gets results through fat loss hormone manipulation. The keys to successful weight loss is knowing the individual and providing the necessary tools to be successful. Society's obesity problem isn't necessarily a result of bad genetics, but rather a result of bad choices and decisions.

Not only does Jayson have an extensive background in weight management, he also has experience in sports nutrition and supplementation. He has published articles on a variety of topics and has consulted with companies, professional teams as well as writers for various articles. Knowing the importance of physiology as it relates to nutrition, Jayson's specialty is working with individuals and getting their nutrition plan as well as their exercise plan set up – so that they not only have an effective individualized plan to meet their goals, but they have a mindset that they will carry with them for the rest of their lives.

CHAPTER 23

HOLISTIC WEIGHT LOSS STRATEGIES

BY STEVE JACK

I have always been fascinated with the human body and what we are capable of, and have been in the health and well-being industry for over 15 years. During that time, I have helped people deal with various weight-loss issues. Early on, I realized that no matter what I recommended, some people just couldn't change shape or lose weight, or they would lose it and then regain it. This used to frustrate me (and them!) and so I began to explore the hidden factors that were keeping people from moving forward and achieving their goals.

Once I began exploring the invisible realm of the mind and the energy system, I realized that these were the secret to unlocking lasting change. Exercise and nutrition were just a part of that. I found that if you have limiting beliefs in your subconscious mind or emotional blockages in your energy system, you will keep repeating the same patterns and no amount of diet or exercise will yield results. Using accelerated reprogramming techniques, I was able to rewire my clients' mind and energy fields to set them up for success with transformational results.

I am about to take you on a voyage of discovery and show you how powerful you truly are.

MIND-BODY-ENERGY TRIAD

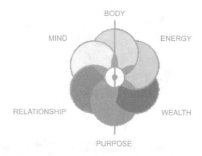

Welcome to my Mind-Body-Energy triad. We will be exploring this as it relates to health and weight loss, although it will have a knock-on effect on all areas of your life. You can't make changes in your relationships, health or work, without making changes to your mind, body and energy field.

The body, mind and energy are all interconnected and you will create the most powerful results when you work on all three simultaneously.

I. MIND: THE CHANGE STARTS HERE

We all see the world in different ways, depending on the beliefs that we have learnt, mainly from our parents, as well as peers, and even the culture in which we live. These beliefs give rise to thoughts, which then go on to shape your world. If you can't steer your mind and thoughts in the direction you want to go, you will literally become stuck in a recurring pattern and wonder why you can't shake your weight.

Your mind literally determines what you do with your body and energy system. It does this by stimulating something in your brain called the Reticular Activating System (RAS), which determines where you will place your attention. The RAS enables your brain to filter and process all the millions of bits of information it receives, thus avoiding overload. However, it scans and codes the information through the lens of your beliefs, distorting or even deleting information so that the world around you reflects what you believe.

This coded information then gets put into your script and is cemented in your subconscious. Just like in the movies your script is the way you play out scenes in your life according to what is written, or in the case of your mind – programmed there.

I once had a client called Anne who just couldn't lose weight, no matter how hard she tried. When we discussed her problems, she admitted that she had fears around relationships, and her underlying belief was: '*If I lose weight, men might find me attractive and start hitting on me, and I don't want the attention.*'

Once we had identified that underlying belief, Anne was able to start changing her thought patterns and she had a breakthrough with her weight loss. It was also an opportunity for her to start addressing her issues with relationships.

Within the developing field of bio-psychology, there are many powerful ways of removing limiting beliefs and literally re-programming the subconscious mind. The one I use the most with clients is Psych-K, which helps to rewrite the software of the past by putting new empowering beliefs in place and changing the printout of the future. To learn more about Psych-k or find a therapist, go to: www.psych-k.com

Once you have embedded new beliefs in your subconscious mind, it is time to start acting on these with the power of the conscious mind. Imagining how you will feel, look and act when you reach your target weight is essential; the mind doesn't know the difference between what is real and what is imagined. This process will also give rise to positive emotions building new neural pathways in the brain. These pathways lead to new behaviour patterns, which are essential for weight-loss.

Here are some practical ways in which to do this:

- Buy a journal and write down your target weight and how it feels, e.g., what you look like, what you are doing, etc. Write this in the present tense as though it has already happened and you have achieved the outcome you want.
- Create a vision board and put it somewhere you can see it everyday. Cut out images, words, diagrams and photos and make a collage to remind you of what you are trying to achieve. You can find out more about vision boards at: http://www.visionboardsite.com

Once you have begun to harness the power of your mind on your weight loss journey, you can start to explore the ways in which you can help your body.

II. BODY: IF YOU DON'T LOOK AFTER YOUR BODY WHERE ELSE ARE YOU GOING TO LIVE?

Hippocrates, the ancient Greek physician and one of the outstanding figures in the history of medicine, stated, "Let food be your medicine and medicine be your food."

Losing body fat and getting your health back on track requires nutrition and exercise. And what you eat and drink affects your energy levels, muscles and even your cells.

Our food supply has been compromised with chemicals and pesticides which interfere with our bodies' biological, magnetic, and electrical signaling systems, all leading to faulty processing in the cells. To counteract this, you need to eat preferably organic food in its natural state. You'll be amazed at the impact this will have on your health and body shape.

THE ELIMINATION DIET

To start off, I recommend going on an elimination diet for 14 days. If you cheat (even once) you must start again. These first 14 days are enough to eliminate the toxins from your system and reset your hormones.

At the end of 14 days have 1 cheat meal, then another cycle of 5 days followed by a cheat meal. Having the cheat meal is important as it makes your body react to excess sugars and releases a hormone that stimulates fat release. It also creates a psychological break from your food plan and helps keep you on track.

WHAT TO ELIMINATE?

The following foods are the major triggers that will mess with your hormones and ensure you hold onto your fat.

(A). WHEAT AND GLUTEN

Modern day processing techniques mean that wheat is devoid of nutrients. Both wheat and gluten (oats, rye etc) can be difficult to digest and slow down the metabolism.

(B). DAIRY (EXCEPT EGGS AND FULL FAT LIVE YOGURT)

Pasteurization and homogenization take out most of the enzymes in dairy products removing the goodness and making them hard to digest.

(C). SUGAR

Sweets, fizzy drinks or anything ending in 'ose' on a food label are highly processed and play havoc with blood sugar levels. They lead to the release of insulin, a fat storage hormone, which converts any excess sugars to body fat.

(D). PROCESSED FOODS

Anything packaged or pre-cooked (including white bread and white pasta) is not only devoid of nutritional content, but includes artificial flavorings and other chemicals.

(E). RED MEAT

This is hard to digest and this can slow down your metabolism and affect your overall digestive processes. It is also very acidic. Once you have achieved your goals, consider having it just once a week.

(F). LOW FAT PRODUCTS

Pretty much all low-fat products have had all the nutrients and good bacteria removed and replaced with SUGAR. It is much better to buy, for example, full fat yogurt which contains the necessary bacteria and enzymes needed for the breakdown and digestion of food.

(G). CAFFEINE

Caffeine gradually wears down your adrenal glands meaning that you have massive energy fluctuations and need 'quick fix' sugary foods that further disrupt your blood sugar and increase fat storage. If you avoid the above foods, you'll find that you don't need caffeine to get you through the day.

(H). ALCOHOL

This is high in calories, for example a glass of wine (250 ml) contains 160 calories, contains no nutrients and increases acidity in the body.

BENEFICIAL FOODS TO ADD

High protein diets based on red meat and dairy are a disaster for the human organism and create a high acidity, low oxygen diet in which cancer and other diseases thrive.

Eat foods that are nutrient dense such as leafy green vegetables (raw or lightly steamed). You also need plant-based protein at each meal such as beans, legumes, lentils, quinoa, chickpeas, tofu and tempeh. These provide all the essential amino acids you would usually obtain from meat, with spirulina being a super food containing all the amino acids you need.

If you struggle to follow a vegetarian diet, then have fish or chicken once a day only.

Also include some nuts and seeds in your diet, as well as extra virgin olive oil and raw coconut oil. These will provide the good fats that you need, which will help speed up your metabolism.

If you follow these nutritional guidelines you will begin to feel amazing after a few days, and the metabolic conditioning will give you extraordinary amounts of energy.

WATER – IT'S WHAT YOU'RE MADE OF

All cells in the body are surrounded by water, so ensuring we consume enough water is vital for health. Most of us are dehydrated without knowing it and drinking enough can help you to keep mentally alert and energetic. You should aim to drink around 3 litres a day; remember that tea and coffee (apart from herbal) don't count! You can even add lemon juice or supergreens (see below).

Our water supply (like our food) has been compromised; there are around 300 toxins found in tap water residue, including fluoride and chlorine. If you can afford it, have a reverse osmosis system fitted. If not, then consider a filter jug or at the very least bottled water. Water will clean up the quality of fluid in your cells and seriously kick-start your metabolism.

SUPPLEMENTS: ADDITIONAL BENEFITS FOR THE BODY

I am not a fan of protein powders or meal replacements. My goal is to make your cells as healthy as possible and I recommend the following:

1. Sodium Bicarbonate with freshly-squeezed lemon juice:

You can buy this very cheaply from supermarkets and it is extremely effective at alkalizing the blood stream and kick-starting your metabolism. Take it first thing in the morning on an empty stomach.

2. Greens Powders

    Wheat or barley grass or any mix of Greens or Supergreens mix are packed with chlorophyll which oxygenates and alkalizes your bloodstream giving you a massive energy boost. I recommend adding these to some water and drinking 2-3 litres a day.

3. Omega 3

    Every single cell in the body is made of fat, and the body requires these so-called essential fatty acids, as it cannot produce them. It is essential to take supplements/flaxseed oil, particularly if you are overweight as your body won't give up any of its fat unless it gets enough in other ways.

4. Spirulina

    Spirulina is 65-71% complete protein, compared to beef's 22% protein. The algae is a source of all eight essential amino acids, as well as chelated minerals, natural plant sugars, trace minerals and enzymes. It is easily assimilated by the body and is also rich in chlorophyll. You can take it in capsule or powder form before meals to get your required protein.

5. Lugol's Iodine

    Iodine is essential for regulation of the thyroid gland and for your metabolism to function normally. Take a couple of drops in a glass of water once or twice a day. If you are on any medication always do this in consultation with your GP.

EXERCISE: JUMP STARTING YOUR METABOLISM

Exercise plays a fundamental role in the weight loss journey, but it needs to be the right kind. Many people don't lose weight because they don't do the right activities. For example, doing 30 minutes of medium-intensity exercise on a treadmill or cross-trainer will increase your metabolism, but it quickly returns to normal. You need to create a metabolic after-burn which keeps your metabolism high for another 48-72 hours. This means that you keep burning calories.

In my experience, the most effective way to achieve this is by merging resistance training with very high-intensity interval training (rather than the slow and steady continuous type). This means that the heart rate goes up, then drops down to a lower level, before going back up again. I call this entire process metabolic conditioning, as it shakes up the metabolism causing it to accelerate and aid weight loss.

The following programme is one that I recommend to many of my clients. If you can complete 3 lots of 40 minute sessions per week you will achieve dramatic results. It includes exercises with a versatile piece of equipment called the TRX, which you can use at home or in the park. You can find more details on my website (www.steve-jack.com). Alternatively, you can substitute TRX exercises with free weights. You alternate the TRX/free weights with high-intensity cardiovascular exercises such as burpees or shuttle runs. Please go to my website to see demonstrations of all these exercises.

I recommend doing each of the following sequences three times taking a two minute break between each one:

Exercise	Reps/time
Sequence One:	
TRX Chest Press	45 seconds
TRX Low Row	45 Seconds
Burpees	15
Sequence Two:	
Giant Step Ups	20 each side
TRX tricep extension	45 seconds
Shuttle runs	6 cones 5 metres apart (100%)
Sequence Three:	
TRX Shoulder retraction	45 seconds
TRX Roll Outs	45 seconds
Lateral step and get down/get up	20 reps

There are other metabolic conditioning workouts on my website (www. steve-jack.com). I suggest that you select three workouts per month and do one once a week. Start with the beginner's exercises and see if you can progress to the more advanced programmes.

III. ENERGY: IT'S ALL ABOUT THE FIELD

My hero, Albert Einstein, said that 'The field is the sole governing agency of matter.' This means anything that is created in the physical world in the form of matter, first comes from or originates in 'the field'. This is because all intentions originate from this field, such as your weight loss goals. In other words, you need to have an intention to lose weight before you can manifest this at a physical level. As a human being, you also have an energy field or aura, which is part of the universal energy field and connects to your environment and to your body.

I have explored this energy field in greater depth with my mentor, ex NASA scientist Dr Barbara Brennan, and have learnt that, over time, we develop unhealthy blocks, which clog our energy field. These often arise from past emotional traumas or painful experiences. As a result we develop limiting beliefs to protect ourselves, which can then prevent us from losing weight or achieving other goals.

There are many ways to clear the energy field. You can work with a certified energy healer (listings can be found on Barbara Brennan's website http://www.barbarabrennan.com/welcome/find_a_graduate.html). Working with energy is very powerful and you need to work with someone who knows what they are doing.

Emotional Freedom Technique (EFT) is another method for shifting energy blockages. It is a simple, yet powerful process that involves tapping your meridian end points, whilst repeating the phrase: "Even though I am... ." For example, "Even though I am overweight, I deeply and completely love and accept myself." Or you could tap on specific issues you are dealing with such as: "Even though I am addicted to chocolate I deeply love and respect myself."

You can find more information and an EFT therapist at: www.eftuniverse.com. I have had great success with this in clearing emotional eating disorders, chocolate addictions and many deeper issues which prevent people from losing weight.

CONCLUSION: WEIGHT-LOSS IS HOLISTIC

I hope that I have awakened you to the different aspects of successful weight-loss and the importance of working simultaneously with the mind-body-energy triad. In my experience you can achieve breakthrough results in this way. Consider exploring these different modalities and open your eyes to a whole new world. You'll be amazed at just how powerful you are!

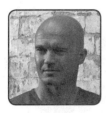

ABOUT STEVE

Steve Jack is a thought leader, speaker and facilitator in health, fitness and well being, with a background in Physical Education, Psychology and Energy Healing. He is considered an expert in health, well-being and performance. For over 18 years he has been working with clients helping them to achieve breakthrough goals in health, well-being, weight loss, and sports performance.

He is a regular on the Professionals Conference circuit having presented in over 20 countries around the world. His business development sessions are changing the way Club Owners and Personal Trainers think about health and wellbeing. Steve helps Club Owners find solutions for increasing secondary spending in their facilities by providing innovative products and training.

Steve writes regularly for a number of international print and online publications, including Mens Health, and is the featured presenter on an online video for well-being and fitness websites. An accomplished speaker and facilitator, Steve has the rare ability to move people in his workshops, and inspires action for those who are ready for change. You can find out more about Steve at www.steve-jack.com

CHAPTER 24

WHERE TO BEGIN WHEN YOU WANT TO LOSE 140LBS+

BY JULIA KNIGHT

The twenty-stone lorry driver ordered egg and chips accompanied by a huge latte and followed with chocolate cake and cream. Several bars of chocolate, an ice cream and a second latte were then purchased in the motorway service area shop before returning to the cab. At just 5'2 and 280lbs this was one seriously overweight lady. And this was me…

Having struggled with my weight for years and having spent far too much money on every new diet product that promised quick-fix results, I was still losing thirty pounds then gaining sixty. Exercise was just not in my vocabulary. I was the typical yo-yo dieter who had written several volumes of the book of excuses, and had some well-crafted reasons as to why I had 'failed' yet again. Every amazing weight loss was swiftly followed by an even bigger gain, and then the following Monday signalled the start of the next 'miracle' diet.

I couldn't visit service areas and expect to find healthy food. I was extremely lucky if they had a jacket potato left. 'Healthy option' is not a phrase they understand. If you have ever been into a motorway service area in the UK, you will know that I'm not exaggerating.

Fitness-wise, nipping down to the gym after work was not an option. I was sleeping in the cab at a service area, a truck stop, or in a roadside lay-by. This is the sort of life-style that makes putting on weight and getting lazy extremely easy. There is an abundance of unhealthy, but quick food on offer, hardly any healthy alternatives, no access to fitness facilities and every excuse in the book to keep getting fatter! I kept telling myself that it was impossible to get a grip of my ever-increasing waistline under such difficult circumstances.

The times when I did take action, I would have a large latte first thing in the morning, continue to drink coffee all day, and then have a toasted cheese sandwich, chocolate muffin and two chocolate chip cookies in the evening. I'm not just guessing here – that is exactly what I would have. These foods were readily available and I thought that as I hadn't eaten anything all day, this was an acceptable method of weight loss.

I was actually doing untold harm. I was starving myself every day. I was functioning on caffeine, and then overloading with sugar and fat all in one go. My body would have interpreted my actions as an indication that there was a problem getting regular nutrition, and would have made various adjustments in order to preserve my life. It stopped sending hunger signals and slowed my metabolism down so that I used my fat stores more slowly. Then, when I ate, it stored the fat away so that I could continue to function in the perceived current emergency. It would also have started to cannibalise my muscle tissue so that it conserved the fat for as long as possible, and this in turn would slow my metabolism down even more. Of course, at first I lost weight, as I was consuming fewer calories than I was using – but as my body adjusted so that I used less energy to compensate for the lack of proper nutrition, I stopped losing weight, lacked energy and assumed that I needed to consume even less. This was not sustainable, and eventually, when I started to eat normally again, I put on the weight I had lost, and more. This is because my metabolism was now slower. Our body is an amazing machine that can do incredible things in order to preserve life, and abusing it with yo-yo dieting is totally unnecessary and ultimately destructive.

I'm now 140 lbs lighter, seven dress sizes smaller. I'm stronger, leaner, fitter and a qualified and successful Personal Trainer. So how did I get from there to here?

At a time when I had yet again lost a large amount of weight, and was then steadily finding it all again, I was taken in hand by a Personal Trainer. I learned that losing body fat, changing my shape and getting fitter and healthier, was within my reach.

The problem is that just the word 'diet' implies that there is an end to the new regime. The diet is often restrictive, tortuous, sometimes unhealthy and therefore unsustainable. You are setting yourself up to regain any losses before you even begin. You have to change your habits for life; a longer, healthier life.

There is an absolute plethora of information on diet and fitness. There is an excess of advice on how to get the body you want, and the explanations get more and more technical and almost always are in conflict with the next or last article that you read. There's a lot of discussion about macro-nutrients, what should be eaten with what, the percentages of carbohydrates, fats and protein that should be consumed. No wonder we end up feeling more confused!

When you have a large amount of weight to lose, this information just serves to make the task look far more complicated than it is. Get yourself comfortable with healthy and nutritious eating, and start to get more active. When you only have a few stubborn pounds to lose or want to sculpt your new body, then you can start getting technical!

So, you're ready to go, but how do you get started? Where is that first step? Say goodbye to all those negative thoughts and start here:

1. Make the decision. Focus. Don't get side-lined by any new diet fad or what you've heard from your mate's mate, or read in the latest celebrity magazine. Be single-minded, determined, and drive forward with your plans. Nothing can stop you getting a better body.

2. Inform everyone that may be affected by your new plans. Include those that you eat with or cook for, those that you go out with, people that you work with who may question why you're

having an *americano* instead of a *latte*. Inform them of your resolution to change your eating plan and ask them for their support. If you let people in, and ask for their assistance, you get far more support than if you try to go it alone. This also makes you accountable. People will ask how you are doing, and will see the results.

3. Count everything! Calorie counting is a good way to get used to the amounts and types of food that you can eat. You won't always have to count everything, but to start with, it will be your guide. When you are very overweight, you don't tend to get, or respond in the normal way to hunger signals. You've either never stopped eating long enough to get hungry, or been on such a severe diet that you learn to ignore them. So relying on your hunger signals when you start on a healthier eating regime may not work – this is where calories will help. Losing weight is very simple: Consume fewer calories than you use. So, add up all your calories for a normal 'non diet' day. Everything includes little extras like biscuits or mints served with coffee, the bits you eat from the kids plates as you clear the dishes, **all** drinks except plain water – EVERYTHING!!! Write it in a book or on a piece of paper, and record it at the time. Don't try to remember it later – that never works.

4. Now you need to work out a sensible daily allowance. If your 'normal' calorie intake is more than 1,700, then simply reduce that by 500. For example, 2,500 calories will become 2,000. Reducing your calories by 500 per day should lead to a weight loss of 1-2lbs per week, which is a safe and sustainable amount to lose. Be patient! Losing more than that every week can mean your body is using lean muscle instead of fat for energy, so you will be defeating the object. In the first few weeks you may well lose more than this as you release water stored with energy sources. This is completely normal. Never drop your calories to less than 1,200 per day; again, this will be counter-productive. If your normal intake is already less than 1,700 and so cannot be dropped by 500, then you can drop the calories to 1,200, but will need to create the full deficit by using more energy. Use the activity guidelines to assist you.

5. EAT BREAKFAST! This is of major importance, and is NOT optional! Even if you haven't eaten breakfast for twenty years, you start now. After having no fuel all night while you were sleeping, your body needs breakfast. If you don't supply energy, it will slow your metabolism in order to conserve energy, to get through until the next mealtime. Don't skip it! Eat 5-6 small meals per day rather than 2 or 3 bigger ones. This regulates your blood sugar, avoids dips in energy and reduces stress on your digestive system. Include fruit, plenty of vegetables and lots of water.

6. Make wise decisions when faced with a choice – go for the lean meat or fish over a pie, choose a fruit dessert instead of a chocolate one, opt for a tomato-based sauce, not a cheese or cream one. The guidelines are really simple, and will make a huge difference to your health as well as your shape and body composition. Don't forget that all drinks that are not plain water must be accounted for. Alcohol has almost as many calories as fat! Count the milk used in your drinks, avoid sugary fruit juices and soda's wherever possible. It all adds up…

7. MOVE! The basic recommendations from ACSM for people aged under 65 and with no known health issues or indications are as follows:

Moderately intense cardio for 30 minutes a day, five days a week. Or, vigorously intense cardio for 20 minutes a day, three days a week PLUS eight to ten strength training exercises, doing eight to twelve reps, twice a week.

Moderately intense means training hard enough to raise your heart rate, produce sweat, but still be able to hold a conversation.

In order to lose weight or create more of a deficit in your calorie intake, you may need to increase the time (30-60 minutes). If you are very new to exercise, break the time down into ten-minute blocks throughout the day until your stamina improves. If you are a beginner, start with more gentle activities like walking or swimming. There are many Internet websites where you can find out how many calories a particular exercise uses, depending on your own weight. ***Always consult your physician before starting a new exercise programme.***

8. Keep a record of your progress: Weigh yourself **once** a week. Use the same set of scales, in the same place, wearing the same clothes, and as close to the same time of day as you can, (first thing in the morning will give far greater accuracy). It doesn't matter too much whether the scales you use are accurately calibrated, as it is the loss that you are measuring. Take a few measurements (chest, waist, hips, upper arm, and thigh). Again, use the same tape measure, at the same time of day and wear the same clothes, if any. Don't check your measurements too regularly, maybe every 4-6 weeks, or if you have a week when you haven't lost any weight. Sometimes you may lose inches instead of weight. Take some photos, in your underwear or swimwear when you start, then take some more every 4-6 weeks. This way, you have plenty of tools to chart your progress and spur you on.

9. There are *no* excuses. I thought I had all the excuses under the sun, but once you make that decision, they become minor irritations that you *can* find a way around. I started to take a supply of healthy foods with me in the cab so that I would always have something available. My other essential was my mobile gym, i.e. my trainers! You can always find somewhere to run or walk. Even parked up on the M25 I could run around the lorry park. There really are no excuses, only your own self-made obstructions.

10. Persist! Losing excess fat is one of those things that you have control over. No one else can do it for you, but you absolutely CAN do it for yourself.

To re-cap: Starting to eat healthily should be sustainable and easy to fit into your life-style. Diets that mean that you can't eat out or eat with the rest of the family will never work for long. You don't need pills and potions, and fad diets will eventually make *you* fatter, and *their creator*, richer.

When you have lost a good percentage of your surplus weight, then you can start thinking about refining your shape and losing the last few stubborn pounds. By then, you will already be comfortable with healthy eating, be more active and may even find that you don't need to do anything else but maintain your new figure.

Don't just read about it. The sooner you take action, the sooner you will see the results. You don't need luck, just resolve, determination and single-mindedness. GO!

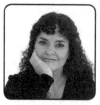

ABOUT JULIA

Julia Knight is a Personal Trainer based in Nottingham, England. She is the proprietor of Fit-Nav Personal Training, which offers one-to-one sessions as well as local bootcamps.

Julia specialises in weight loss, calling on her personal experience of dealing with the associated problems of obesity, and has a level three qualification in Weight Management and Nutrition. She holds a Diploma in Personal Training, is an Advanced Fitness Instructor, Kettlebell Instructor, Thump boxing instructor, holds additional qualifications in Active Ageing and is a Biomechanics Coach.

In her spare time, Julia practices the martial art of Shindo Jinen Ryu, and is also a keen drummer. Her ambition is to continue building on the ever-growing reputation of Fit-Nav and to help more and more people to see that changing their body shape and fitness levels are within everyone's reach, with the right guidance.

CHAPTER 25

MISSION: METABOLISM

DISCOVER HOW TO FIX THE SEVEN DEADLY WORKOUT SINS TO ACHIEVE METABOLIC BREAKTHROUGH

BY BJ GADDOUR

A s a former fat kid and disgruntled owner of a naturally slower metabolism, I have made it my life's mission to help other people like me achieve metabolic breakthroughs to dramatically improve body composition, performance, and overall health.

I am the proud owner of MISSION: METABOLISM BOOTCAMP in Milwaukee, WI. The program features 30-minute express metabolic workouts for busy people who are looking to physically empower themselves to take on any challenges that life throws their way.

What follows is a culmination of years of research and trial and error to produce rapid and lasting weight loss through cutting-edge metabolic training that only requires a 90-minute commitment each week.

First, you will learn what metabolism is.

Next, you will discover how to fix the seven deadly workout sins that plague most fitness enthusiasts in order to achieve metabolic breakthrough.

Lastly, you will be empowered with a one-month, done-for-you, home/travel fitness program to dramatically accelerate your metabolism, burn the stubborn belly, hip, and thigh fat, and build lean, sexy muscle all over your body.

Alright baby – time to crank up that metabolism!

WHAT IS METABOLISM?

Metabolism is the sum of all chemical processes that take place in the human body to sustain life. Many people are born with slower metabolisms that make them prone to weight gain. Other people, known as lucky ____ (fill in the blank), are born with faster metabolisms and seem to have no problem being lean regardless of their activity levels or dietary habits … yeah, I hate them too, ha! ha!

Though metabolic rate is largely determined by genetics, there are various ways to increase metabolic rate (the speed of your metabolism) though exercise, nutrition, and supplementation. For our purposes, we will focus solely on the metabolic impact of a properly designed exercise routine.

THE 7 DEADLY WORKOUT SINS… AND HOW TO FIX THEM TO ACHIEVE METABOLIC BREAKTHROUGH!

DEADLY WORKOUT SIN #1 – Performing daily body part workouts

One of the longest running inside jokes within the fitness industry is the fact that Monday is "international chest day" where most gym-goers will do endless sets and reps of bench presses and chest flies, until their boobies "burn so good" and swell – as if being nipped by a swarm of 'ginormous' mosquitoes.

We can thank the drug-abusing bodybuilding world for the concept of training one body part per day for best results. If you open the typical bodybuilding magazine, below is a great example of a training program you might come across (or some variation of this):

Monday- Chest
Tuesday- Quads
Wednesday- Back

Thursday- Hamstrings
Friday- Triceps
Saturday- Biceps
Sunday- Calves

Please keep in mind that when you take a cocktail of anabolic perfor-mance enhancing agents, just about anything you do will result in less fat and more muscle– not to mention a host of deadly side effects and the possibility of growing a tail (anything is possible, you know).

The reality is that training your whole body more frequently will result in bigger strength and muscle gain, greater fat loss, and more metabolic boosts than training each muscle group once per week– and the science supports this.

In a recent study at the University of Alabama, researchers had two groups of men perform two different strength-training programs with the same total training volume (sets and reps) for each muscle group. However, one group split the work across three total body workouts while the other group trained each muscle group separately one time per week. They dis-covered that the total body workout group gained five additional pounds of lean muscle mass compared to their body-part training counterparts.

Lastly, it appears that it's best to wait about 48 hours before performing your next total body workout. In multiple studies at the University of Texas Medical Branch in Galveston, researchers determined that muscle protein synthesis was elevated for up to 48 hours after a resistance train-ing workout before it returned to normal. Performing another total body workout with less than 48 hours of recovery may not allow for adequate muscle repair thus impairing performance.

THE FIX: For busy people looking for the biggest bang for their fitness buck, best results will be achieved with 3 total body workouts per week, with ideally 48 hours between workouts – to maximize muscle growth and recovery.

DEADLY WORKOUT SIN #2 – Performing marathon workouts lasting 60 minutes or longer

I'm not sure what it is about our society that thinks its cool to do things for an incredibly long period of time. There's no better example of this than the typical college student who brags to his or her friends about pulling an all-nighter to cram for a final exam. In reality, best results would have been achieved by spreading out all of that studying over the course of the entire semester in order to achieve true and lasting knowledge, rather than simple and useless short-term memory. I'd be lying if I said I've never procrastinated before myself as I'm literally writing this chapter the day before its due date -- but don't tell my editor, wink!

Fitness is no different. What do most people who want to lose weight do? They either sign up to run a marathon and/or join a gym to do endless hours of long, slow, boring cardio on a treadmill, elliptical, bike, or step machine.

On a side note, if I ever see you "getting your cardio-on" while reading a magazine or checking your email I will 'slap you in the mouth' and have you arrested for being a hopeless moron.

A landmark aerobic training study from the International Journal of Sports Nutrition determined that 45 minutes of steady state aerobic training (think long, slow, boring cardio) performed 5 days per week had zero effect over dieting alone when it came to weight loss— that's 45 hours of activity for nothing! However, the lack of results wasn't solely due to the length of the workouts, but also the low-intensity nature of these workouts.

In addition, long, drawn-out workouts have diminishing returns and create a negative hormonal environment in our bodies. That's because during one-hour plus exercise bouts our body enters survival mode and releases a catabolic stress hormone called cortisol that both causes muscle loss and results in unwanted fat gain in trouble spot areas.

According to the National Strength and Conditioning Association (NSCA), anabolic, muscle-building hormones like testosterone are maximized in about a 30-minute high-intensity workout window. It is at about the 45-minute mark that anabolic hormones begin to fall as their catabolic counterparts, mainly cortisol, simultaneously begin to rise.

THE FIX: Shorter, more focused and intense workouts produce better results than 'one hour plus' marathon sessions. If you have to workout for longer than 30-45 minutes to feel satisfied, then you probably weren't working hard enough in the first place, or you were committing some form of the other deadly workout sins.

DEADLY WORKOUT SIN #3 – Using single-joint isolation exercises that address only one plane of movement

When we discussed *Deadly Workout Sin #1*, we mentioned the disgraceful practice of training each muscle group one time per week. Well, to make the matter even worse, lots of fitness enthusiasts will comprise these body part workouts with useless single-joint isolation exercises that often take place in only one plane of movement.

Single-joint, isolation exercises involve the use of only one joint at a time. Classic examples are leg extensions and leg curls (only involve the knee joint) and biceps curls and triceps extensions (only involve the elbow joint). Though these single-joint, isolation exercises may result in a better "pump" or "burn" in a specific muscle that makes it feel more effective, it doesn't mean that they are providing the optimal muscle-building stimulus when compared to their multi-joint, compound counterparts.

Multi-joint, compound exercises involve functional movement patterns that occur in the real world across multiple joints at the same time. This results in greater total muscle activation and heavier loading and subsequently greater calorie burning, fat loss, and muscle growth.

For our purposes, there are six foundational movement patterns that comprise the ultimate total body metabolic workout:

1. **HIP-DOMINANT:** Any exercise that primarily targets your posterior chain (glutes, hamstrings, and spinal erectors), and involves the flexion, extension, rotation, adduction, and abduction of the hips. In addition, lower body exercises where your torso is bent forward more than 45-degrees are best classified as hip-dominant. The exception to this rule is for any exercise where the upper body is NOT actively involved like a hip extension. Classic hip-dominant exercises include deadlift, step-up, hip extension, and swings.
2. **PUSH:** Any exercise that primarily targets your chest, anterior and medial shoulders, and triceps, and involves a pushing pattern in either the horizontal or vertical plane. Horizontal pushing exercises involve pushing a load away from your

torso as if your torso was upright while performing them.
Classic examples include push-up and chest press variations.
Vertical pushing exercises involve pushing a load in an
upward or downward direction relative to an upright torso.
Classic examples include dip, vertical push-up or overhead
press variations.

3. **KNEE-DOMINANT:** Any exercise that primarily targets
   your quadriceps and involves the flexion and extension of
   your knees. In addition, lower body exercises that actively
   involve your upper body and where your torso is vertical or
   bent forward less than 45-degrees are best classified as knee-
   dominant. Classic knee-dominant exercises include squat and
   lunge variations.

4. **PULL/SCAPULOTHORACIC:** Any exercise that primarily
   targets your lats, posterior shoulders, upper and mid back,
   scapulothoracic joint, biceps and forearms and involves
   a pulling pattern in either the horizontal or vertical plane.
   Horizontal pulling exercises involve pulling a load towards
   your torso as if your torso was upright while performing
   them. Classic examples include rowing and Y, T, W, L, I raise
   variations. Vertical pulling exercises involve pulling a load in
   an upward or downward direction relative to an upright torso.
   Classic examples include pull-up, pull-down, high pull, and
   bicep curl variations.

5. **PILLAR-INTEGRATED SHOULDERS, HIPS, AND CORE:**
   Any exercise that primarily targets your shoulders, hips, and
   core. The primary objective is to train spinal stabilization in all
   3 planes of movement including anti-flexion, anti-extension,
   anti-lateral flexion, and anti-rotation. Classic examples include
   front, side, and back pillar or plank variations. Pillar movements
   also include functional, ground-based rotational exercises like
   chopping variations.

6. **TOTAL BODY:** Any exercise that integrates any combination
   of the aforementioned movement patterns or simultaneously
   calls upon your upper and lower body. The total body nature
   of these exercises also results in maximum heart rate elevation
   and the optimal fat-burning, muscle-building stimulus. Classic
   examples include squat to presses, swings, and explosive

olympic lifting variations like cleans, snatches, jerks, etc. In addition, traditional cardiovascular locomotive and plyometric exercises like running, leaping, hopping, skipping, bounding, jumping, shuffling, etc. also fit under this category.

In a study at Ball State University, researchers determined that additional isolation exercises for the arms had no additional benefit in terms of arm strength and hypertrophy (muscle growth). One group did four compound upper body exercises (like presses and rows) in each workout while the other group did the same four exercises plus some extra biceps curls and triceps extensions. Since they both achieved the same results it appears that single-joint, isolation exercises have minimal if any benefit.

So now that we know the importance of training movement patterns (not body parts) with multi-joint, compound exercises, let's not forget about the importance of incorporating exercises that occur across multiple planes of movement.

Too often people perform exercises in only one plane of movement, typically the sagittal plane that encompasses movement up-and-down and front-to-back. The classic exercises that fit the bill here are bench presses and squats.

However, movement in life and athletics occurs in three planes of motion: sagittal, frontal, and transverse. Sagittal plane movements occur up and down and front to back and divide the body into left and right halves. Frontal plane movements occur side-to-side and divide the body into front and back halves. Transverse plane movements occur in a rotational manner and divide the body into upper and lower halves.

Let's use the lunge as an example. A forward lunge takes place in the sagittal plane, where a lateral lunge takes place in the frontal plane, where a rotational lunge takes place in the transverse plane. Performing lunge variations in all three planes of movements best ensures optimal strength and muscle gains plus proper muscular balance, which in turn improves posture and bolsters injury prevention.

I should add that performing exercises in free space is ideal (also termed "free weights"). Machines limit movement to a fixed path and do not properly engage your body's key stabilizers which will put you at risk of injury outside of the gym.

THE FIX: Employ functional multi-joint, compound movement patterns that address all three planes of movement for maximum muscle growth, fat loss, and metabolic spikes.

DEADLY WORKOUT SIN #4 – Using low-intensity work periods lasting 2 minutes or longer to burn fat

This one is mainly for all of the ladies out there- and I'm not about to sing a Michael Bolton or Marvin Gaye song here… unless of course, the price is right.

Women have the relentless tendency to perform endless hours of cardio and if they do use weights, they tend to use loads that are so light that they might as well not even bother — so small that they can barely be seen with the naked eye.

Heck, most guys out there have a hard enough time gaining muscle. Now factor in that women have 15-20 times less testosterone than men do and the answer is clear. In other words, women never have to worry about gaining too much muscle -- it would require freakish genetics and loads of drugs to even come close. Using heavier loads will just result in greater calorie burning, a faster metabolic rate, and a tighter, more toned and athletic physique.

One of the biggest myths in fitness is the concept of the fat-burning zone. It all started in 1993 when researchers at the University of Texas determined that lower to moderate intensity activity burnt the greatest amount of fat for fuel. In addition, peak fat oxidation (burning) appeared to occur at 65% of aerobic capacity. This is basically the exercise equivalent of conversational cardio or a power walk or slow jog.

However, we've already seen in the study mentioned earlier that 45 hours of aerobic training had zero effect on weight loss over dieting alone, so we know that a power walk or slow jog will just not cut it.

Furthermore, though lower intensity exercise burns proportionately more fat than high-intensity exercise, high-intensity exercise burns more total calories per minute, and thus still burns a similar amount of total fat during exercise as its lower-to-moderate intensity counterpart.

The fact of the matter is that high-intensity exercise is scientifically proven to burn nine times more body fat than ordinary exercise per unit of effort. Plus, it's not about how much fat you burn during your workout that's important. The harder you exercise, the more carbs you burn for fuel, and this allows you to burn more fat during rest periods and in the hours and days between your workouts – for maximum total body fat burning.

For the best real world example of which style of training is best for lean muscle gain and fat loss, just look at the body of a sprinter versus the body of an endurance athlete. Sprinters are not only more muscular but actually have a lower body fat percentage than endurance athletes. Though I've seen lots of overweight distance runners and walkers in my day, I have never seen an overweight sprinter. That has to count for something and again the science supports this theory.

In the Gibala Study, researchers collected a bunch of college students who were in good health but not participating in any athletics. One group rode a bike at a sustainable pace for 90-120 minutes. The other group performed 20-30 seconds of cycling at maximum effort followed by 4 minutes of full recovery and they repeated this sequence up to four to six times for a total of 18-27 minutes. Each group exercised three times per week for two total weeks. In the end, they discovered that both groups achieved identical improvements in endurance, even though the high-intensity group had only exercised for six to nine minutes – while it took the low-intensity group five hours to achieve those same results! I know, crazy, right?

What's even crazier is the fact that the high-intensity group had greater weight loss than their low-intensity counterparts. According to the head researcher Martin Gibala, the "rate of energy expenditure remains higher longer into recovery" from high-intensity interval training.

There's something special about high-intensity anaerobic (without oxygen) work periods of 30-60 seconds. First of all, they are glycolytic in nature meaning that they burn muscle glycogen, the sugar stored in your muscles, at optimal rates. The more sugar you burn during your workouts, the more body fat you will burn in the hours and days between your workouts.

Second of all, research has shown that maximum hypertrophy, or muscle growth, occurs when performing exercises with heavy loading and a time-under-tension lasting 30-40 seconds. At a rep speed of two to three seconds per rep that comes down to the classic bodybuilding rep range of eight to 15 reps per set. More muscle gain means greater metabolism which means more rapid and lasting weight loss.

Lastly, high-intensity anaerobic work periods of 30-60 seconds also create the optimal hormonal environment for fat loss by releasing hormones knows as catecholamines (mainly adrenaline). This surge of adrenaline mobilizes body fat, particular in the stubborn areas like the abs and lower back for men and the hips and thighs for women.

Interestingly enough, resorting to shorter and even higher-intensity work periods of 20 seconds or less, actually causes a greater catecholamine release that leads to even greater fat mobilization during the workout. On the other hand, not as much glycogen will be depleted with these shorter work periods, thus resulting in less fat being burnt at all other times of day. However, employing shorter, more intense work periods with incomplete rest periods will deplete your phosphagen stores (ATP-CP), and force your body to start using more sugar for fuel (this is beyond the scope of this chapter).

In general, I believe it's a fair trade off. Plus, the best interval training protocol is the one you haven't done in a while, if ever. In other words, I recommend incorporating a wide variety of work periods ranging between 30-60 seconds or less for maximum fat blasting and metabolic disturbance and to keep your body guessing.

The bottom line is that intensity is the only thing that truly makes your body change. If you take one thing away from this chapter, I hope it is this!

THE FIX: To burn fat and skyrocket metabolism 24/7/365, employ high-intensity work periods lasting 30-60 seconds or less to deplete muscle glycogen stores during your workouts – in order to burn more fat fuel when resting and at all other times of the day.

DEADLY WORKOUT SIN #5 – Performing straight sets of a single exercise

It takes about three to five minutes following intensive exertion for your body to completely recover and get ready for another bout of maximum effort, without any significant decreases in performance. In traditional weight training, if you're performing three sets of 10 reps, that means that it would take a minimum of 10-15 minutes to complete your first exercise in your workout, putting you 'on track' for one of those 'one hour plus' marathon sessions that we already know is not optimal.

However, there is a very simple way that we can maintain peak intensity while allowing for full recovery: perform alternating sets of non-competitive exercises. This is also referred to as circuit training.

Typically it takes a trainee about 30 seconds to complete 10 reps of a given exercise at a controlled tempo of three seconds per rep. Previously we outlined that there are six basic movement patterns that make up any sound training plan with each movement pattern emphasizing a different region of the body. So let's build ourselves a 'killer' six-exercise metabolic circuit, where we allow for about 15 seconds of rest and transition between exercises, and a 60-second rest and transition at the end of the circuit to re-group:

1. Hip-Dominant Exercise @ 30 seconds on, 15 seconds off
2. Pushing Exercise @ 30 seconds on, 15 seconds off
3. Knee-Dominant Exercise @ 30 seconds on, 15 seconds off
4. Pulling Exercise @ 30 seconds on, 15 seconds off
5. Pillar Exercise @ 30 seconds on, 15 seconds off
6. Total Body Exercise @ 30 seconds on, 15 seconds off

Let's examine the beauty of what we just did here:

- In approximately five minutes, the circuit format allowed us to perform all six exercises that comprise a whole body workout, where in the straight sets format, it took us the same amount of time to complete one set of a single exercise
- By alternating between non-competitive exercises in a circuit format, we are able to achieve maximum intensity while allowing for a full 5-minute recovery by the next time we repeat that same exercise
- In only 20 minutes, we can complete four rounds of this whole body circuit and be done for the day, while we'd just be starting our second set of the second exercise in straight-set format

Clearly the circuit training format is by far the most time-efficient approach, and it also has many other of the key variables for metabolic training in place, such as: high-intensity work periods, short and focused 20-minute workouts, short rest periods, total body workout, etc.

I believe circuit training is the foundation of any solid metabolic workout. Let's take a look at two breakthrough scientific studies that support what I've seen in the real world:

BURN OVER 500 CALORIES IN 20 MINUTES: In a recent study by the University of Southern Maine, researchers discovered a more accurate method of estimating calorie burn from weight training than had been used previously. They discovered that a weight training circuit burned 71% more calories than previously thought. In fact, an eight minute circuit burned somewhere between 159 and 233 calories which breaks down to about 20-28 calories per minute.

ELEVATE METABOLISM FOR UP TO 38+ HOURS POST-WORKOUT: In a study by the European Journal of Applied Physiology, researchers determined that a 31-minute circuit training protocol of three compound, multi-joint movements significantly elevated metabolism for 38 hours post-workout – at which point they decided to stop tracking. This metabolic afterburn was due to a couple of factors. The first is due to increased tissue turnover due to the need to build and repair the microtrauma to the muscles after high-intensity exercises. The second is due to increased Excess Post-Exercise Oxygen Consumption (EPOC) due to the oxygen debt created by high-intensity anaerobic exercise.

From a personal standpoint, when I was young and stupid football player, I used to workout for two to three hours at a time using the straight set format. It was always incredibly mentally draining to know that half of my day would be eaten up every time I worked out. However, I had all of the time in the world to workout so I took advantage of that. Strangely enough, I had a lot of extra body fat for someone who was working out for several hours a day— that's weird, right?

Now that I'm not as young and a little less stupid (I think), and I am the owner of several fitness companies, both online and offline, the only workouts I currently have time for are metabolic circuits that have me in and out in 30 minutes, and on with my busy, hectic days. Today I maintain a single-digit body fat percentage and it's all due to these circuits and sound diet that emphasizes protein, produce, and water every couple of hours.

The choice is yours-- get better results in less than half the time or take hours of your precious time to get frustrating results. Well, I guess it's not much of a choice after all.

THE FIX: If your goal is maximum results in minimal time, employ alternating sets of non-competitive exercises each and every time you workout. Metabolic circuit training is by far the best way to get into the best shape of your life in 30 minutes or less so you can get on with your very busy day.

DEADLY WORKOUT SIN #6 – Using long rest periods of 2 minutes or more between exercises

How many times have you seen this happen in the gym:

A big, burly, meathead of a man lays down to grunt out a couple reps of heavy benches presses where the bar bounces off of his chest like a basketball, while his butt leaps off of the bench with his lower back more extended than Gumby.

Then he racks the weight and goes and grabs a swig of water or chugs a vat of a protein drink.

A couple minutes, pass and now he's watching some highlights on Sports Center with a few of his meathead buddies.

A couple more minutes pass, and now he's molesting some good-looking cardio queen with his eyes.

Finally, five to seven minutes after he completed his last rep on the bench press, he's ready to start his next set.

More likely than not, this guy will take several hours to complete his work-out at this pace. Clearly, this is not the most efficient way to exercise.

Now, if your goal is maximum strength and power, then three to five minute complete recovery periods have their place.

But chances are, if you're like most of the general population, you couldn't care less about how much you can bench or squat and are more focused on having the lean, muscular build of a Men's or Women's Health model.

In other words, most people can afford to lose some fat and gain some muscle and the key to doing so is to maximize training density. Density describes the amount of work completed per unit of time. Density also happens to be the biggest primer for fat loss, because the more work you can complete in the same amount of time or less, the leaner and more muscular you will be.

How do we accomplish this? We do so by reducing our rest periods between exercises. According to the NSCA, shorter rest periods lasting 30-60 seconds or less resulted in the greatest growth hormone response. Growth hormone is one of the most powerful fat-burning and muscle-building hormones in your body.

Look no further than the world famous Tabata Study for the fat-burning, metabolic-boosting benefits of high-intensity work periods combined with short rest periods. In this groundbreaking cycling study, researchers discovered that a mere four minutes of a 20 -10 interval protocol (20 seconds of maximum effort followed by 10 seconds of rest) provided greater fat loss and conditioning than 60 minutes of steady-state cardio.

Now, one of the problems with this study is that in the real world most people aren't able to perform multiple bouts of max effort for the same exercise with short rest periods (in fact, most of the elite cyclists in the study couldn't complete all four minutes of the 20-10 protocol because it was too intense).

However, by employing a circuit training format where you perform alternating sets of non-competitive exercises, we can maintain the high-intensity work periods in conjunction with the short rest periods, as in the Tabata study.

Furthermore, I have personally found this 2:1 negative work to rest ratio (in this case, 20 seconds on, 10 seconds off) to be unreal for rapidly improving fat loss and fitness for my campers, and for my own personal workouts (more on this later).

THE FIX: Employ short rest periods of 30-60 seconds or less between exercises, in order to maximize training density and the growth hormone response from exercise – for maximum fat loss and metabolic acceleration.

DEADLY WORKOUT SIN #7 – Performing the same fitness routine for six weeks or more

This one is pretty straight forward – if you perform the same workout routine day-in and day-out, week-in and week-out, your body will stop changing and you will hit a dreaded plateau.

The classic example of this can be seen in any 'run of the mill' gym or health club. On day one, after your sign a contract where you pay money to use somebody else's equipment, you'll meet with a "personal trainer" on day one – who probably is wearing some cute little jacket that says "personal trainer" on it (I'm convinced the reason for this is because some personal trainers may actually forget what they do for a living – too much protein on the brain). Then he or she will teach you how to use all of the machines (don't get me started on machines), and will then recommend doing a circuit of three sets of 10 reps for each body part every time you workout.

Now keep in mind that if you are sedentary and haven't exercised in years (if ever), absolutely anything you do in the gym will elicit a positive response. If you exercise with heavier loads, your body will respond by gaining more muscle to accommodate the new training demands. If you employ shorter rest periods between sets while maintaining the same total work output, your body will respond by improving conditioning and melting unwanted body fat. If you perform a new exercise altogether that challenges your body in a very unique way, your nervous system will quickly figure out how to master this movement, resulting in increased performance.

The human body is a smart and efficient machine, and will quickly adapt to any training plan that you throw its way. Within the first two to three weeks of any new training program, you will notice the biggest improvements in your performance and physique. However, the human body is constantly striving for homeostasis and efficiency, and after performing the same program for about four weeks there are diminishing returns.

That's why it's critical to change-up your fitness routine every month. By simply tweaking a couple of variables in your training plan, like your exercise selection, exercise order, work periods and rest periods, etc., you provide a new stimulus that will force your body to change and prevent dreaded physique plateaus.

Now, don't get me wrong here – we always perform the same movement patterns in every training program because they are foundational.

However, there are lots of different exercises that fall under the same movement pattern category that we can cycle between. New exercises require more mental and physical energy to perform – thus burning more calories and causing a greater metabolic disturbance, and this is exactly the type of stimulus your body needs to break out of any fitness rut.

The best example for this is the push-up, since there are literally hundreds of push-up variations. We pretty much do some sort of push-up variation every workout, but by constantly switching up the type of push-up we're using, there is always a new stimulus that keeps the body changing. Plus, the better you get at one type of push-up, the better you get at all of the others.

In addition, let's not forget about the mental component here. The brain needs variety and performing the same routine for extended periods of time will not only decrease performance, but will also lower your motivation to workout. So you'll start skipping training sessions here and there, and then all of a sudden, you'll find yourself back at square one—sitting on your butt, twiddling your thumbs, while watching an infomercial about this incredible new waist belt that will give you the flat tummy of your dreams… all for only four easy payments of $19.95, so it can sit under your bed and collect dust, before your dog uses it as a new chew toy.

I have personally programmed for thousands of people online, and I have worked with hundreds of campers in the trenches for many years. What I've discovered is that if I simply swap in new exercises and move to a different interval training protocol every three to four weeks, I can constantly keep their bodies changing and performance continues to improve. Not to mention the fact that their motivation to workout remains sky high with every new challenge I throw their way.

My camps operate on a three weeks on, one week off schedule-- I've found this to be the sweet spot for the typical busy person in their 20's through 50's. We work very hard for three weeks, trying to keep pushing the envelope each subsequent week by providing a gradual progressive overload. Then we employ an active recovery week to allow for mental and physical regeneration, and to prevent overtraining or unwanted injury. Then we start a new program altogether, and we wash and repeat like clockwork. The results have been simply amazing.

THE FIX: Switch up your fitness routine each and every month to prevent dreaded weight loss and performance plateaus. Employ new exercises and different work and rest periods (or interval protocols) to constantly provide a new stimulus that your body must learn how to adapt to.

PUTTING IT ALL TOGETHER

Now that we've outlined the seven keys to metabolic breakthrough, let's put it all together in a readily-usable metabolic training program so you can start cranking it today!

A **Metabolic Workout** features a total body workout that employs high-intensity work periods with short rest periods in an alternating set or circuit format, that combines the muscle building benefits of resistance training with the cardiovascular benefits of cardio training. The result is a killer bootcamp-style workout that will supercharge metabolism for up to 48 hours post-workout, build lean muscle, blast belly fat, and get you into the best shape of your life with only three 30-minute express workouts per week.

If you recall from the Gibala study, it was determined that 30-second maximum effort work periods followed by four minutes of rest for 20 straight minutes resulted in identical fitness improvements and greater weight loss than 90-120 minutes of aerobic training. By building a circuit of non-competitive exercises, we can allow for this same full recovery, and thus peak intensity, by the next time we return to the original exercise.

Furthermore, we demonstrated that 30-second max effort work periods provide both a big-time metabolic boosting muscle-building stimulus plus deplete your body's sugar stores at optimal rates, forcing it to burn more fat during recovery periods and in the hours and days between workouts.

In addition, I outlined the Tabata study which found that a 2:1 negative work to rest ratio found in a 20-seconds on, 10-seconds off, four-minute high-intensity interval training protocol resulted in greater fat loss and conditioning than 60-minutes of steady state cardio. Short rest periods increase training density, and produce a growth hormone response that boosts whole body fat-burning and lean muscle gain.

However, I have found that for most de-conditioned beginners, 20-second work periods do not allow for a sufficient amount of time to adequately perform enough muscular contractions for optimal results, and that 30-second work periods are a much better time frame to best accommodate people of all fitness levels. Using this 2:1 negative work to rest ratio for 30-second work periods means that we would employ a 30-15 interval protocol with 15 seconds of rest between exercises.

Ladies and gentlemen, without further ado, below is what I've discovered to be the ultimate metabolic experience...

30 – 15 SIX-EXERCISE METABOLIC CIRCUIT – 20 MINUTES: Alternate between 30 seconds of work and 15 seconds of rest for each exercise in the following 6-exercise circuit followed by a 60-second rest and transition between circuits. Perform up to 4 total rounds for a 20-minute total body workout.

Station#	Exercise Variation
1	Hip-Dominant Variation
2	Push Variation
3	Knee-Dominant Variation
4	Pull Variation
5	Pillar Variation
6	Total Body Variation

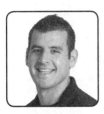

ABOUT BJ

BJ is a former fat kid and a self-proclaimed "work in progress" who has made every mistake in the book when it comes to health and fitness in his own life. Upon graduating from the world-renowned Amherst College as a double major in economics and sociology, BJ found he wanted nothing to do with either career path. As a former college football player and a life-long workout junkie, he discovered his calling was to empower others to forever change their bodies and lives for the better. BJ has a unique ability to translate his own personal failures into remarkable successes for the people he works with.

BJ is widely considered to be the world's leading fitness boot camp expert. He owns and operates *MISSION: METABOLISM BOOTCAMP* in Milwaukee, WI, which features 30-minute express metabolic boot camp workouts for busy professionals looking to optimize body composition, performance, and overall health. To learn more please visit:

http://MissionMetabolismBootcamp.com

BJ is also the Co-Creator and Fitness Director for *Workout Muse*, a fitness music and media production company. Workout Muse specializes in custom interval training workout music soundtracks and smartphone fitness solutions. To learn more and to download some free samples, please visit:

http://www.WorkoutMuse.com

BJ is also passionate about helping fitness professionals all over the world make more money by helping more people, in order to solve the raging obesity epidemic crippling our world. He lectures nationally as a Perform Better presenter for his expertise in fitness boot camp program design and business systems.

Downloading Your Digital MISSION: METABOLISM Bootcamp-To-Go

As a special thank you for purchasing this book and reading my chapter, I have put together a cutting-edge, one-month done-for-you training program taken straight out of my MISSION: METABOLISM BOOTCAMP using the aforementioned 30-15 Metabolic Circuit Training protocol to jump-start your results.

In conjunction with a proper nutrition plan that focuses on protein, produce, and water every 2-4 hours, you can expect to drop a dress or pant size in 21 days.

I am sure you are used to seeing exercise pictures and written descriptions when being provided with a workout program. However, exercises are truly dynamic in nature and are best shown and taught via video and that's how we'll be doing it.

To instantly download your complimentary home/travel fitness program, featuring instructional workout videos complete with a proper warm-up and cool-down, custom interval training workout music soundtracks that tell you exactly what to do, and cheat sheets outlining all of your workouts, please visit the following website:

http://www.workoutmuse.com/totalbodybreakthrough

How "Metabolic" is Your Workout?

Please reference the chart below to assess the current metabolic status of your fitness routine. If your main goal is to improve your body composition (burn body fat and build lean muscle) and revamp metabolism then you absolutely must structure your workouts to fall under the metabolic breakthrough column.

	Metabolic Rut	Metabolic Breakthrough
Training Split	Daily body part workouts	3 total body workouts per week with ideally 48-hours between workouts
Length of Workout	60 minutes or more	30-45 minutes or less
Exercise Selection	Single-joint, isolation exercises that address only 1 plane of movement	Functional multi-joint, compound movement patterns that address all 3 planes of movement
Exercise Intensity	Low-intensity work periods of 2 minutes or longer to burn fat	High-intensity work periods of 30-60 seconds or less to burn sugar
Rest Periods	Long rest periods of 2 minutes or longer	Short rest periods of 30-60 seconds or less
Exercise Order	Straights sets of a single exercise	Circuit Training: Alternating sets of non-competitive exercises
Periodization	Perform the same fitness routine for 6 weeks or more	Progress to a new fitness routine every 3-4 weeks

CHAPTER 26

NUTRITION SUPPLEMENTS

BY JAYSON HUNTER

There's No Magic Pill, but …

There are hundreds, if not thousands, of nutritional supplements on the shelves today. Some are good, and some are, frankly, garbage. How are you to determine what's what, and if you should even be taking supplements?

Well, I'm here to advise you that there are supplements you should be taking. I've done the research for you, so you'll know which brand to get, what you should take, and why.

During the 12 years I've worked as a Registered Dietitian, I've seen more awful supplements than I've seen good ones. Based on this experience, I know how to weed out the bad products in favor of good ones. And I have my finger on the pulse of research that shows what's most effective in this area.

In this chapter, I share with you which supplements are most effective for helping you lose weight. So without further ado …

1. FISH OILS

Supplements with fish oil are an excellent way to get important Essential

Fatty Acids (EFA), such as DHA and EPA. Remember, Essential Fatty Acids such as these may help prevent cancer, heart disease, depression and more. And they can't be produced by the body – we must get EFA from outside sources like food and supplements. This is why we call these fats "essential."

OTHER BENEFITS OF TAKING FISH OIL:

- Improves concentration and memory
- Provides protection for cell membranes
- Aids in healthy nervous system function
- Improves cholesterol
- Supports a strong immune system
- Relieves PMS symptoms
- Promotes heart health
- Fights the damaging effects of aging
- **Encourages FAT LOSS!**

Let's discuss that last benefit in greater detail. Not only is fish oil containing EFA important for general health and disease prevention, it's a great way to enhance your fat-burning efforts. That's not to say it's a magic fat-loss pill. Sorry, there's no such thing. However, you can take comfort in knowing that recent studies have shown supplements containing Essential Fatty Acids may have miraculous results.

The enormous health benefits of Essential Fatty Acids have been known for some time, but what's almost startling is the recent research uncovering its weight-loss benefits, as well. In May 2007, a study published in the *American Journal of Clinical Nutrition* reported that a test group incorporating Essential Fatty Acids into their weight-loss plan lost more body fat than all the other test groups in the study combined!

While science hasn't pinpointed exactly why Essential Fatty Acids improve weight loss, I have several theories:

- DHA has been shown to prevent the conversion of pre-fat cells to fat cells, as well as kill pre-fat cells before they become permanent fat cells.
- Fish oil has the ability to increase both the clearance of chylomicrons (a certain type of fat cell) and fats following a meal. This may have a positive effect on fat usage for energy.

- Fish oil can "artificially" decrease heart rate, thus increasing the level of exertion you need to reach a desired exercise intensity. Simply put, you burn more overall calories when exercising.
- Fish oil increases oxidation of fats within fat cells. This means your body burns more fat as energy instead of storing it.

Considering the overwhelming clinical research pointing to the advantages of EFA supplementation, most weight-loss enthusiasts should be incorporating it into their nutritional plans. I am so convinced of this product's benefits, I recommend it to every one of my clients. The brand and product I recommend is Prograde Nutrition's EFA Icon at http:// www.getprograde.com/essential-fatty-acid.html

2. POST-WORKOUT RECOVERY DRINK

Post-workout shakes provide a foundation for accelerated fat loss and recovery after exercise. Research shows that consuming a specific mixture of carbohydrates and proteins enhances recovery of muscle nutrient stores.

How does this affect you? Significant glycogen (i.e., carbohydrate) storage greatly reduces the time it takes your body to recover from exercise. This means you are able to make the most of every workout and burn more calories for fat loss.

In addition to the right kind of carbs, consuming protein immediately after exercise is essential for repairing muscle tissue that has been damaged from exercise (don't worry, this "damage" is a normal part of exercise). Protein also provides the essential amino acids needed to repair muscle tissue so it's ready for your next workout.

Carbs and protein are vital for repairing and preparing your body for the next workout. You should consume a recovery drink within 1 hour of exercise – the sooner, the better. This is the most critical period for replenishing muscle glycogen and amino acid absorption, so you increase lean body mass and burn more calories for weight loss.

If you pass up the proper post-workout nutrition, your exercise performance may suffer the next time you work out. And you may even lose muscle along the way if you don't replenish glycogen and protein quickly.

So what's in a good post-workout supplement? An effective workout recovery drink supplies a blend of high-quality proteins; quick-digesting carbohydrates; free-form amino acids; vitamins; and, finally, essential minerals, including antioxidants to help maximize post-workout recovery. To optimize your training, improve your recovery time, and accelerate fat loss and muscle growth, consume a post-workout drink as part of your training routine.

A GOOD POST-WORKOUT DRINK CONTAINS:

- A formulated 2:1 blend of quick-digesting carbohydrates to protein.
- Protein that's made up of Whey Protein Isolate, which has a concentration higher than 95% protein. Whey Protein Isolate has a very high biological value, meaning it's great for before and after workouts because it's so readily digested, absorbed and used by the body.
- Carbohydrates that consist of dextrose and maltodextrin to facilitate quick absorption and utilization by your muscles.
- The essential B vitamins necessary to provide energy to your cells. This starts the recovery process or fuels cells with energy for upcoming activity.

3. WHOLE-FOOD MULTIVITAMIN

WHY DO PEOPLE NEED TO TAKE A MULTIVITAMIN?

Consistent use of multivitamins and other key supplements can promote good health and help prevent disease, according to a comprehensive new report released by the Council for Responsible Nutrition (CRN).

The report found that ongoing use of multivitamins (preferably those with minerals) and other single-nutrient supplements (like calcium or folic acid) had a positive and quantifiable impact on everything from strengthening elderly patients' immune systems to drastically reducing the risk of neural tube birth defects, such as spina bifida.

This news has relevance for people trying to lose weight, as well. Based on the American Medical Association's recent evaluation of the medical literature, the association recommends Americans consume a one-a-day multivitamin in order to promote general health. Doing so will help you meet your goal to look better and *feel better*.

HEALTH BENEFITS OF TAKING A MULTIVITAMIN:

- Provides complete daily nutritional supplement foundation
- Provides essential vitamins, minerals, enzymes, amino acids, phytonutrients and whole-food concentrates for optimum health that's unique to women
- Alleviates vitamin deficiencies
- Increases energy levels
- Helps maintain healthy metabolism
- Whole-food base aids assimilation of nutrients
- Supplements any lack of nutrients (e.g., fruits and vegetables) in your diet
- Replaces nutrients depleted by stress

4. WHY ALL THESE PROTEIN POWDERS?

You see, Protein is where it's at.

Check out these two little known facts about protein:

1. Protein requires more calories to digest than carbs or fat. This is called the "thermic effect of food." In other words, your body uses more calories to digest protein than other nutrients. Pretty sneaky, huh?
2. Protein provides satiety. That's a fancy way of saying you feel fuller for longer when you eat protein.

Good sources of Lean Protein come from foods such as: Fish, eggs, poultry, lean beef...

But some people have trouble eating enough protein each day. Some people would like it to be more convenient for them.

If that's the case with you then I have VERY good news. There are protein powders on the market that are pharmaceutical quality whey protein.

You see, not all protein powders are created equal. You want to look for protein powders that deliver these qualities:

- Unparalled purity through low-temperature micro-filtering

- Is naturally sweetened with Stevia
- Contains at least 4 grams of branch chained amino acids per serving
- Mixes instantly with just a spoon
- Enhances absorption and digestion via lactase and Aminogen digestive enzyymes

There are more expensive protein powders on the market for a reason. The reason is they use the standards I listed above. Higher quality means higher cost so don't settle for a $10 jug of protein from the local store because you will not be paying for quality at that point. I recommend this protein powder here: http://www.getprograde.com/protein-powder.html

YOUR NEW LIFESTYLE AWAITS

I suggest you track your body fat and body circumferences every 3 weeks. Doing so allows you to effectively evaluate whether you need to modify your eating or exercise habits.

Be aware that your progress will change as your transformation continues. At first, you'll see a lot of progress quickly. As you become thinner, that progress will slow down a little. Don't get discouraged and, please, don't obsess over numbers on the scale.

Remember, with proper diet and exercise, you're adding lean muscle at the same time you're losing fat. If you lose 3 lbs of fat, yet gain 3 lbs of muscle, the number on the scale won't budge. But you'll look and feel a whole lot better. And your old dresses, skirts, shirts and jeans will fit a lot looser ... In fact, you'd better plan to buy a new and improved wardrobe.

Well, what are you waiting for? If you haven't already, it's time to start your dramatic body transformation. If you've already used the contents of this book to reach your initial goals – congratulations! You have the rest of your life to enjoy a healthier, slimmer body.

No matter what stage you're at, following the strategies in this book means an exciting new lifestyle is part of your future! Enjoy.

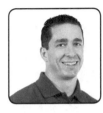

ABOUT JAYSON

Jayson Hunter RD, CSCS is the author of the Carb Rotation Diet as well as the Director of Research and Development for Prograde Nutrition. He is also a best selling author and contributor for the book: Big Ideas for Your Business.

He has also been featured on CBS, ABC, FOX and NBC to discuss his very successful Carb Rotation Diet program.

His nutritional programs have helped thousands of clients successfully lose weight and create permanent lifestyle changes. Jayson's method of eating and nutritional programming gets results through fat loss hormone manipulation. The keys to successful weight loss is knowing the individual and providing the necessary tools to be successful. Society's obesity problem isn't necessarily a result of bad genetics, but rather a result of bad choices and decisions.

Not only does Jayson have an extensive background in weight management, he also has experience in sports nutrition and supplementation. He has published articles on a variety of topics and has consulted with companies, professional teams as well as writers for various articles. Knowing the importance of physiology as it relates to nutrition, Jayson's specialty is working with individuals and getting their nutrition plan as well as their exercise plan set up – so that they not only have an effective individualized plan to meet their goals, but they have a mindset that they will carry with them for the rest of their lives.

CHAPTER 27

ABS UNCRUNCHED

– HOW TO GET A FLAT STOMACH WITHOUT EVER DOING A SINGLE CRUNCH

BY SCOTT COLBY

Who here wants to lose belly fat?

Now who here wants to lose belly fat without:

- Spending any more money on a gym membership
- Spending any money on any fancy fitness equipment
- Wasting your time driving to the gym or waiting in line to use a machine
- Doing 2 hour workouts, or even hour long workouts
- Ever doing another crunch again!

Does this sound good to you?

HINT: Everyone should be nodding and raising their hands right now.

Good. I'm glad we're in agreement.

Now, before we move on, do you mind if we get the serious stuff out of the way first? If you have excess belly fat, you should be afraid. In fact you should be downright scared. Of course, when you look at your belly in the mirror, a feeling of disgust and shame may be crossing your mind because you can't stand how ugly your belly looks. Guys are worried about how they'll look when they take their shirts off at the beach, or in the bedroom, and women are worried about looking hot in their bikini or skinny jeans.

But this is not the kind of scared that I'm referring to. Unfortunately, having excess belly fat is not all about looks. It's actually a serious health issue too. While we know it's dangerous to have excess body fat, scientific research has shown that having excess fat in the abdominal area is even more dangerous and can lead to serious health problems.

There are two types of fat that you have in your abdominal area. The first type that covers up your abs from being visible is called subcutaneous fat and lies directly beneath the skin and on top of the abdominal muscles.

The second type of fat that you have in your abdominal area is called visceral fat, and that lies deeper in the abdomen beneath your muscle and surrounding your organs.

Both subcutaneous fat and visceral fat in the abdominal area are serious health risk factors, but science has shown that having excessive visceral fat is even more dangerous than subcutaneous fat. Both of them greatly increase the risk, your risk, of developing heart disease, diabetes, high blood pressure, stroke, sleep apnea, various forms of cancer, and other degenerative diseases.

So losing your belly fat should be one of your top priorities, not because you'll look and feel a lot better (although that's a nice side benefit), but because you'll be at a lower risk for all types of illnesses and diseases.

OK, now that we got the serious stuff out of the way, can I share a story with you?

Did you know I used to be just like you?

That's right. I used to hit the gym after work about 4 days a week. My workouts usually consisted of weight training one or 2 bodyparts each time I went to the gym. You know, chest and back one day, biceps and triceps another day and shoulders and legs on the third day. My weight training workout usually took about an hour.

Then, if I felt like it, I usually got on the treadmill for a walk or a jog for about 30 minutes. And then I would end the workout by going to the corner with all of the mats and doing various types of crunches for about 5-10 minutes. You know the ones – regular crunches, twisting crunches, crunches with my legs in the air, crunches with my legs in a frog position…and any type of crunch I could think of.

I'm guessing that your workout is similar to mine. Or worse yet, maybe you reverse it and do an hour of cardio and only a few minutes of weight training. Either way, do you still have extra belly fat? I know I did. I mean I really wanted six pack abs, but no matter how hard I worked out, the elusive six pack abs remained just that – elusive.

I thought I was eating healthy most of the time too. Cereals and orange juice for breakfast, wheat bread and lunch meat for lunch, reduced fat wheat crackers for snacks, and sometimes a frozen dinner or I'd cook dinner myself. I usually treated myself with a dessert after dinner.

This was all to no avail. I had a fairly lean body but just couldn't get rid of my excess belly fat – that is until I got smart.

Being in the fitness industry, I decided to take matters into my own hands. I sat down and interviewed some of the top fat loss and abs experts in the world. I looked at the research to find out what workouts worked best to reduce belly fat. And I put it all together into a system that I tested on myself and a few select clients.

And guess what happened?

I finally got six pack abs. My clients' got rid of their ugly belly fat and reduced their waist size by a lot.

And…lucky for you, I'm going to share my 6 Flat Belly Secrets with you so that you can finally get rid of your ugly belly fat too!

FLAT BELLY SECRET #1

You don't need to spend 1-2 hours in the gym to get a flat stomach.

As a fitness professional, I've heard all the excuses in the book for skipping a workout: too busy, gym is too crowded or too far, don't have my workout clothes or sneakers, it's too hot or cold outside. And the list goes on and one. But by far the #1 excuse I hear over and over again for skipping a workout is, "I don't have enough time."

Well let me break it down for you: there are 1,440 minutes in a day. Can you spare 20 minutes or less and dedicate that time to exercising and reducing your belly fat? If you said "no" you should just stop reading this chapter right now. If you said "yes", then great! That will still give you 1,420 minutes to get the rest of your stuff done during the day.

FLAT BELLY SECRET #2

You don't need any equipment to lose belly fat.

Bodyweight workouts are extremely effective at helping you burn belly fat and get an all around hot body. They are the most convenient form of workouts and can be performed anywhere – in your home, in the backyard, in a hotel room, at a gym, etc., so you're more likely to stick to your routine.

But there are biomechanical reasons why bodyweight movements are so effective. You see, in life we use our body as one full segment, like sitting down, reaching for something on a shelf, turning around, chasing your kids, or any of hundreds of other movements.

Your body should be trained mimicking these movements to best cope with the demands of daily living and sports. Machines at the gym can make you stronger but they isolate individual muscles too much and that's not how your body is designed to work. Remember, we said that you use your body as one full segment. If you isolate muscles when you train, this can lead to imbalances and overuse injuries.

FLAT BELLY SECRET #3

You don't need to do any crunches to get a flat stomach.

There are a few problems with crunches. First, crunches isolate one muscle group – the abs. Remember we said that in everyday living, the body works as one unit and it's better to train it as such.

Second, when you do crunches, you are lying on your back on the ground for part of the time, so your abs are relaxed and not even working during a portion of the crunch.

Third, your abs play a critical role in stabilizing your spine (not flexing it) and should be trained as such. During crunches, your abs are helping to flex the spine, not stabilize it.

And finally, crunches are not an intense enough exercise to where you'll be burning fat calories. So for these reasons, crunches should be eliminated from your workout program.

FLAT BELLY SECRET #4

Exercises that work your abs the entire time, such as exercises in a standing, push up or plank position, are going to work best at flattening your belly and getting your entire body defined and lean.

Exercises that fit this description are squats, push ups and forearm planks.

These type of movements not only train your abs, but, since they are compound movements, they work more than one muscle group at a time. Many of the movements are strengthening movements, which help to build lean muscle in your body which induces a fat-burning effect.

If the exercises are organized in the proper order with little rest between movements, you can simulate a high-intensity cardio effect training in an anaerobic state. This will allow for increased metabolism for several hours after the workout is complete, allowing your body to burn more fat calories.

FLAT BELLY SECRET #5

Incorporate weight-based interval training into your workouts.

Combining your weight training with cardio workouts – full body weight exercises with heavy weights and sprint-based drills inserted continuously into the workout – will help you burn more fat.

A recent study by Davis, et. al., published in the Journal of Strength and Conditioning, examined 2 groups of exercisers. Group A did 60 minutes of resistance training followed by 30 minutes aerobic training. Group B alternated resistance training with a high intensity treadmill sprint (the weight-based interval training group).

Group B showed an almost 10-fold reduction in body fat greater than Group A, and over 80% increase in muscle strength over Group A!

A sample weight-based interval training workout would look like this (see pictures at the end of the chapter for proper technique):

Push Ups x 30 seconds
Squat Jumps x 30 seconds
Close Grip Push Ups x 30 seconds
Squat Thrusts x 30 seconds
Feet Elevated Push Ups x 30 seconds
Mountain Climbers x 30 seconds
Rest for 60 seconds and repeat for 3 rounds total

Another powerful type of training is using Tabata Intervals. Tabata training intervals are 4 - minute intervals, where you perform 20 seconds maximum intensity exercise followed by 10 seconds of rest. You perform 8 straight rounds for a total of 4 minutes.

Dr. Tabata's original study was performed on a cycle ergometer for 6 weeks, where participates exercised 4 minutes a day/3 days per week. The results were a 28% increase in anaerobic capacity and 14% increase in VO2 max in the study participants.

You can try Tabata Intervals with different exercises – keep in mind this may change the focus, e.g., push ups would make it a strength-endurance focus. The intense interval work raises the metabolic rate long after the exercise session is completed resulting in more post-workout fat loss.

Try the protocol with sprinting, jump rope, or bodyweight movements like push ups, squats and squat thrusts.

A simple, but effective sample Tabata protocol would be as follows:

Push Ups x 20 seconds
Rest x 10 seconds
Squats x 20 seconds
Rest x 10 seconds
4 rounds of each = 4 minutes

FLAT BELLY SECRET #6

Count ingredients, not calories. Eat single ingredient foods and foods with as few ingredients as possible.

No matter how much you work out, it won't help much if your diet is out of whack. You should be eating whole, natural foods as often as possible, and get rid of the sugars, processed and boxed foods, as well as foods high in trans fat. Even foods that you might think are healthy, such as cereals and reduced fat crackers, are just as disguised as health foods. Check out the ingredient list. It's a paragraph long and contains lots of junk.

Examples of foods that you should be eating include: eggs, spinach, apples, oatmeal, chicken, turkey breast, sweet potatoes, salmon, almonds, strawberries, blueberries, and walnuts.

So to sum up, to lose belly fat and get a flat stomach, focus on these core principles:

1. Use functional movement patterns similar to daily life with compound exercises, not isolation exercises
2. Train the abs for stability not flexion
3. Include a blend of challenging bodyweight training and interval cardio for maximal fat loss
4. Count ingredients, not calories

STANDARD PUSH UPS – Knees will remain off the ground the entire time (beginners can have knees on the ground). Hands are shoulder width apart. Lower yourself as low as you can while keeping a straight back. Extend all the way up without arching your back.

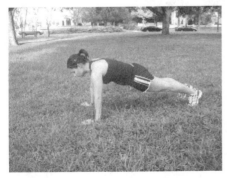 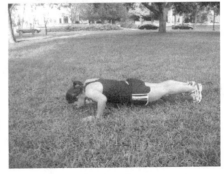

CLOSE GRIP PUSH UP – This variation emphasizes your triceps more than your chest. Your hands are close together, directly underneath your chest. It is a more difficult movement than the standard push up.

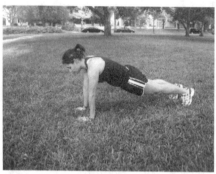 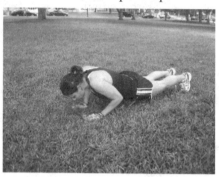

FEET ELEVATED PUSH UP – Placing your feet on a bench makes this push up more demanding, but it also forces you to work your abs as they are stabilizing your body and helping you maintain position.

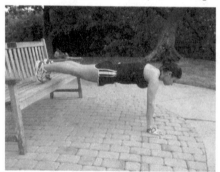 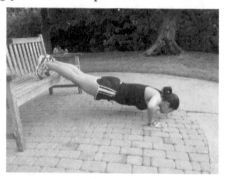

SQUATS: With your feet about shoulder width apart and your arms crossed in front of your chest, drive your hips back and while keeping your weight over your heels, lower yourself as far as you can go while still maintaining a straight back. Return to the start.

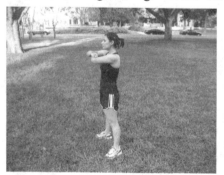 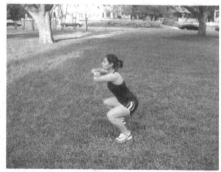

SQUAT JUMPS – Going down into a squat, explode up and jump as high as you can, swinging your arms back. Land into a squat and repeat.

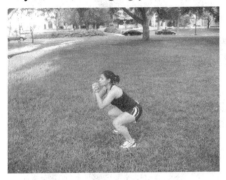 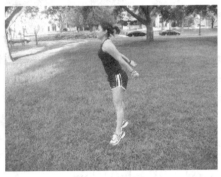

SQUAT THRUSTS – From a standing position, squat down with your hands on the ground. You will then kick your feet back into a push up position. Quickly kick your feet back in and complete the movement by exploding up into the air with a jump and your arms over your head. As soon as you land, go into the next one.

For an added challenge, do one push up while you're down in the push up position before you explode back up.

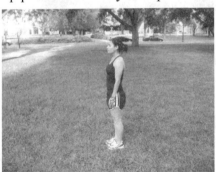 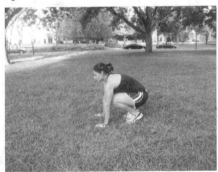

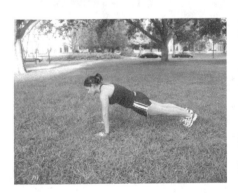 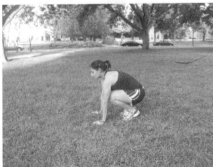

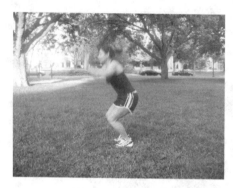 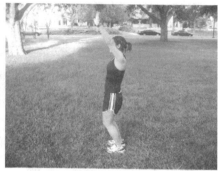

MOUNTAIN CLIMBERS – Begin with your hands on the ground. One leg should be tucked while the other one is extended. With your weight on the balls of your feet, alternate legs back and forth as quickly as possible like you are running in place.

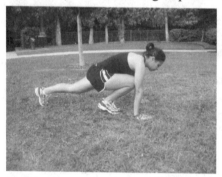 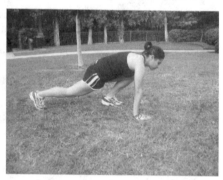

ABOUT SCOTT

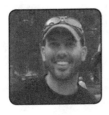

Scott Colby is a certified personal trainer. He holds a Masters degree from the University of Virginia specializing in Biomechanics, and has over 10 years experience in conducting research in human movement.

Scott specializes in helping frustrated and confused men and women finally achieve the toned, tight, sexy body they've always wanted. He has worked with literally hundreds of people – both personally on a one-on-one basis with clients, and in his Women's Only Bootcamps in Dallas, Texas. And that doesn't even include the thousands of men and women he has consulted with and helped in his online businesses, his teleseminars, and his other products.

Scott is an internationally known fitness professional speaker, and he is the author of the internationally popular Abs Uncrunched and creator of the My First Six Pack coaching program.

In addition, he is the owner of AbsUncrunched.com and The AbsExpert.com . Scott is the creator of the online teleseminar series My Ultimate Body Makeover and Amazing Abs Formula, and Mommy Abs Makeover which have helped tens of thousands of people in over 100 countries around the world.

He also founded Her Strength fitness bootcamps for women in Dallas, Texas which he has owned and operated for over 5 years.

Scott's latest venture is his new business, Fitness Adventures USA, providing healthy vacations and active fitness adventures all over the United States.

Scott Colby – The Abs Expert

For a FREE 21 Day Road Map to Fat Loss, please visit:
www.RapidFatLossBlueprint.com

CHAPTER 28

THREE THINGS TO BUILD YOUR BODY NATURALLY

BY TYLER ENGLISH, NASM-PES, CPT, YFS

What supplement can I take for _____?

You fill in the blank, because you yourself have either thought this, or even asked the question, of your trusted "expert."

Not a day goes by where I don't discuss, recommend or consume a supplement. As a fat loss, nutrition and physique enhancement coach, it is a part of my daily grind.

Working with hundreds of clients in a week leaves open the opportunity for me to answer questions regarding proper nutrition, meal planning, meal timing, proper macronutrients, and yes, proper supplementation. Many times my answers shock people who I feel are expecting to hear what they may, or may not have been told, at the local supplement store.

This is an age where everyone, from the local youth athlete to the de-conditioned gym-goer, can step into anyone of these supplement stores and be told, "you need to take this to accomplish that." That makes what I do, and my belief in proper supplementation, even more important for a client or future client.

Now you're more than likely thinking to yourself: What supplements does he take? Before I even begin to tell you how I use supplementation to maximize my health, I want you to understand what I used to believe was the answer to a healthy, strong and muscular physique.

EARLY YEARS: THE EXPERIMENT

I experimented, yes experimented, with strength training or "lifting", as we cool kids called it, when I was in elementary school.

In the basement of my house, my Father, who was an avid recreational boxer when he first met my mother, had an assortment of old plastic weights that were filled with concrete. Well, I just thought this was the coolest thing. The only problem, I had no clue what I was doing. Being a young skinny athlete, I wanted to be bigger and stronger. So I benched, curled, gripped, pressed and tried all types of what I considered strength training movements, in my quest to "get big."

Then, as my years went on, I did what most young children do. I became more consumed with "being a kid" and playing team sports. What I did not realize was that this "experimentation" was only the beginning of what would become the answer to my success in life and business.

Growing up, I was always involved in sports. From the time I could walk, I played baseball, basketball, soccer and wrestled. I don't think a day went by where my Mother wasn't driving me, my sister Tara or my brother Robert, to a practice or a game. It was what we English children did and did it well.

All of my accolades were achieved by my sheer desire to be the best at whatever I did. I was very athletic, super competitive, naturally strong and fast. What I lacked in overall size, I made up in hard work and determination.

Then, it wasn't until I reached my high school years that the "The Weight Room" seemed to be a way of life. Yet again, a few familiar roadblocks popped up in my life. I became consumed with being part of "the *in* crowd" or "partying" and lost my focus for playing sports.

The peer pressure associated with my first two years of high school only gave me time to maintain such a status. Oh, and did I pay for it! It affected my attitude, my athletic ability, my schoolwork and ultimately, my grades.

My sophomore year of high school I weighed a whopping 114 pounds, and through natural growth spurts would only weigh around 125 pounds by my junior year.

Athletic? Yes. An imposing figure on the field of play? Not so much. This would all change.

A good friend, who was a standout on our football team, got me into the weight room on a regular basis. By the start of my junior year, I began lifting weights 5-6 days per week. It became an obsession.

At the start of our senior year, I had grown to 155 pounds of solid, lean muscle. When I showed up for preseason practice, my varsity soccer coach couldn't believe his eyes. Yes, I had packed on close to 30 pounds of muscle in a less than a year, yet I wasn't satisfied.

Besides all the meals I was consuming, I began to read everything I could get my hands on. All I kept seeing were these advertisements for different types of supplements. Their targeted messages regularly called out to me.

"Take *this* to build your muscle mass!"

"Take *that* to increase your lean muscle by 300%!"

Many of these supplements cost $40 – $100 per container. An expensive cost for a mere teenager, but I had a way. Upon starting my senior year of high school I was only playing one sport, soccer, as I had walked away from wrestling and baseball in order to get a job. I had a solid job, working in the warehouse of a successful furniture company. This meant I had money to spend and spend it I did.

On supplements and more supplements!

I was under the distinct belief that one of these powders or pills was going to be the path to the physique I desired. The local GNC became a frequent stop for me. Gold Card Tuesdays were my opportunity to buy the latest and greatest while saving some money.

Even after reading hundreds of online articles about supplements, spending anywhere from $200 to $400 per month on supplements, drinking, swallowing and experimenting with everything from Mass Building Powders to over-priced Natural Testosterone Boosters (mind you, I was 17 and had plenty of naturally occurring testosterone), and the latest and greatest pre- and post-workout drinks over and over again, I still wasn't where I wanted to be.

My friend, the same friend who had helped me get started, told me where he could get us "a cycle" of testosterone. A simple cycle I thought, how hard could that be to do? I thought… I'll be bigger… I'll be stronger, and it will all happen so much faster!

Well, from the start I knew something didn't feel right. My buddy set up the entire process and actually drove us to meet "the seller", who just so happened to be someone we both already knew. The entire situation was just not right.

I mean, does secretly meeting a person in a shopping plaza parking lot to illegally purchase steroids sound right to you?

So he purchased them for us, two cycles to be exact, one for him and one for me. I remember not being able to spend the upfront money on the steroids, because I was already spending so much money on supplements and food, so he fronted me the money. But in my eyes, they never were mine or meant to be mine. Well, he immediately started his cycle and began to see strength and size gains. He would update me almost daily about the changes he was seeing.

Me? I would hide my vial in a secret compartment or hiding place in the dresser in my room. An entire 3 weeks would pass and I would never attempt to administer the steroids. There were days I would come home from school and take it out, stare at it, but nothing would come of it.

Like I said, the whole thing seemed wrong from the start, and the thought of sticking myself with a needle… the thought freaked me out! NO WAY! I was the child who was deathly afraid of getting a flu shot up until middle school! I never came into possession of the 'tool' I would need to administer the drugs, …just the vial, and it would sit there the entire time. After my friend had completed his cycle, he knew I hadn't taken the step. So, I gave him mine to do as he chose.

Did the thought of attempting this again ever cross my mind? I'd be lying to you if I told you no. Even in college I would still buy supplements, only now I became obsessed with finding the "Holy Grail" of the Supplement World.

Despite my early frustrations and experiments, the industry continued to pour out total BS. I would still spend the money on supplements, only now I was stepping over the line of …dangerous. I was in college and began to hear about these things called Prohormones. They were available in most supplement stores and online, which of course, I thought, made them ok.

Still, in the back of my mind I kept thinking that these were too good to be true. They were being marketed as steroid-like results, without the nasty side effects. Even better, they were in pill form. No nasty needles. Initially working in the journalism field in college, I used the skills I had learned. I began researching. I researched everything there was to know about supplements. I found ways to stack and cycle. For a period of 3 months, I experimented with what I thought was the "Holy Grail" of the supplement industry.

I began to see my weight increase, my strength increase and ultimately my muscle mass also. I was weighing in at 206, benching 225 pounds for 23 repetitions, and squatting close to 400 pounds, all at the tender age of 20 years old.

There was a downside. My obsession took control of me. It's all I wanted to do. I remember seeing an ESPN special on these Prohormones and Steroidal Precursors.

Major League Baseball stars were taking them, NFL standouts were taking them.

How bad could they be? I began to see a change in my attitude, my mood and my energy levels. This was after only from 3 months of use! I knew it needed to change.

CREATING A NATURAL LIFESTYLE

Upon graduating from college, I followed my passion into the fitness industry.

I started working as a personal trainer in two gyms. I began to become a research-a-holic. I would read and research everything on the human body, anatomy and physiology, nutrition, fat loss and muscle growth. One aspect I became quite fond of was the effect of proper nutrition and diet on the human body.

I began to change the way I approached exercise, nutrition and supplementation. What I had failed to realize earlier on was that there was a way supplements could help you maximize your body's potential. There is a very healthy, safe and effective way to achieve the physique you desire.

I began to discover the need for essential nutrients, and even though essential nutrients are found in our food, a large portion of the population falls short in their intake of these essential nutrients. Introducing essential nutrient supplements into our daily lives can help develop a healthier population and become a long-lasting strategy for a healthier lifestyle.

THE THREE NATURAL WAYS TO MAXIMIZE YOUR BODY'S POTENTIAL

I'm a firm believer the world revolves in threes – you can agree or disagree. To alter your body composition is no different.

To achieve a lean, muscular, healthy body you need to balance three things:-

1. Nutrition
2. Strength Training
3. Cardio

And yes, in that order of importance.

My clients are made well aware that "you can't out-train a bad diet", no matter how awesome the workout. It also goes without saying that you need the proper balance.

– No matter what 'Diet Plan' you follow, no matter what Strength Training program you perform on a weekly basis, and no matter how much or what type of cardio you perform, there needs to be a consistent balance. Creating a proper caloric deficit will allow you to burn body fat.

– A consistent strength training program will allow you the opportunity to build new lean muscle while adding an increased 'caloric burn' post-workout.

– Cardio, be it interval cardio, metabolic circuit training or steady-state cardio, will aid in creating a caloric deficit by burning excess fat calories from your body.

However, I am not here to tell you how to maximize these three components. No, I am here to tell you the three natural things you need to get fit naturally, and allow you to change your body composition naturally. So by now, I hope you understand that we need exercise. Everyone should understand this, though I get that some choose not to.

In our world, 86% of the population does not exercise yet we can find that 80% of the population is "on a diet." Many of these dieters are willing to take supplements to help speed along their results. It surprises many of my clients, friends and fellow competitors when I explain to them I take nothing more than 3 essential things per day.

1. PROTEIN AND AMINO ACID SUPPLEMENTATION

Your body needs protein in order to build new lean muscle. After all, the ability to build lean muscle will increase your body's overall metabolism – allowing it to become more efficient at burning body fat.

A whole-food based protein source is always recommended, but many times inaccessible in our fast-paced lives. I tell all my clients to remember that a "complete protein source at some point in it's life had a face, a mother, and it could swim or could fly" – meaning that lean meat from chicken, turkey, fish, lean red meat, lean dairy and egg whites all fit in this category.

Complete proteins contain a complete amount of essential amino acids. These essential amino acids are responsible for everything – from our structure, to our enzymes, and to our hormones. Therefore, without the adequate amount of daily consumption, we risk the loss of valuable lean muscle from a negative protein balance.

When it comes to living our lives on-the-go, a protein supplement or amino acid supplement can be a big aid in allowing us to get our recommended daily protein and essential amino acids – by allowing our body to preserve valuable lean muscle.

Studies have shown post-workout that a liquid blend of protein and carbohydrates will absorb into your bloodstream quicker and more efficiently to allow you to recover quicker. This begins the process of repairing, recovering and rebuilding correctly, and at a much more effective rate.

There are numerous ways you can consume a protein supplement. It is preferably my recommendation to use milk, egg, and rice proteins that have a complete Amino Acid Profile and are Non-GMO or a "non-genetically modified organism" meaning that the protein you are consuming is from a naturally-occurring source in nature, and has not been created through genetic engineering. Protein supplements should say "Non-GMO" on them and include no "bovine growth hormone." Our market has recently become flooded with low-grade protein supplements that can do your body more harm then good.

Protein supplements like whey, rice or egg protein can be used as snacks in yogurt, oatmeal, cottage cheese or as a baking ingredient to increase the overall protein value in a recipe. A popular use for protein is following a workout or as a midday smoothie meal replacement, all by adding some fruit with yogurt, almond or rice milk.

Another great source of protein supplementation is the use of Protein and Carbohydrate Workout Drinks. They should contain a mixture of quickly digested and well-tolerated protein and carbohydrate in a ratio of 2:1 or 3:1 carbohydrates:protein. This should be consumed following all high-intensity exercise, when muscle strength and size increases, and an increase in athletic performance is desired, or a Branched-Chain Amino Acids supplement (that contains the 3 BCAAs leucine, isoleucine, and valine) during all high-intensity exercise when fat loss and muscle preservation is the desired result.

2. ESSENTIAL FATTY ACID SUPPLEMENT
(HIGH OMEGA-3 CONTENT)

You can consume your essential fatty acid intake from fatty fish such as salmon, anchovies, sardines and other fish. Though, if you are like me and don't keep fish as a staple in your diet, then the void needs to be filled. In fact, much of the world's available supply of whole-food fish contains levels of environmental pollutants. Therefore it is a better option for us, as healthy individuals, to supplement our essential fatty acid intake with a high quality omega-3 supplement.

Consuming essential fatty acids has been shown to aid in promoting fat loss by supporting healthy blood sugars, supporting heart health, optimal joint comfort and has been shown to enhance mood balance by providing relief of PMS symptoms in women.

When consuming omega-3 fats, the most important are alpha-linolenic acid (ALA), docosahexaenoic acid (DHA) and eicosapentaenoic acid (EPA). Land plant sources such as flax and walnuts are rich in ALA, whereas marine sources like fish oils and algae (the true origin of omega-3 sources for fish), are rich in EPA and DHA – which are recognized as the most beneficial omega-3 fats.

These can be taken daily with meals in doses of 2-3 grams or as high as 6-9 grams of total high omega-3 content (containing at least 30% EPA and DHA) in the form of high-grade fish oil or krill oil, which has been shown to eliminate "fish burps", and krill oil has been shown to improve both LDL and HDL cholesterol. Some other benefits to Omega-3 consumption are better skin, higher sex drive, improved brain function, better recovery, less inflammation, improved cardiovascular health and lower body fat.

3. SUPPLEMENTAL GREENS
AND MULTI VITAMIN / MULTI MINERAL

The average person is deficient in several micronutrients and unless someone is very conscientious about their diet, then a vitamin and mineral or greens supplement is recommended with meals or on days where dietary intake is poor.

I for one have come to realize if you are very conscientious about your diet, then a greens supplement can be more beneficial than that of a multivitamin or multi- mineral. Though, as more people are willing to pop a pill than consume fruits and veggies, the average person will more than likely end up consuming one or both.

I am someone who consumes up to 10 servings or more of fruits and vegetables a day, and I still consume a green food blend high in antioxidants daily. Your frequency can depend on your own personal fruit and vegetable intake. If you feel that your intake is lower, then you will need to take them more frequently.

As for a vitamin and mineral supplement, there are many "synthetic" types on the market that are a waste of your time and money. When purchasing a 'multi' be sure to look for those that are "whole-food based", and that will supply you with the antioxidant capabilities of a greens supplement.

Some other things to look for in a 'multi' are essential phytonutrients, enzymes, amino acids, vitamins and minerals. For those very conscientious about their daily consumption, a healthy diet high in fruits and vegetables aided with a greens supplement is all your body needs in order to get back any deficiencies in micronutrients.

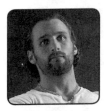

ABOUT TYLER

Tyler English, NASM-PES, CPT, YFS has quickly become Farmington Valley Connecticut's leading Fitness Expert. He is the founder of Connecticut's Most Elite Fitness Program, Farmington Valley Fitness Boot Camp. Tyler is a National Academy of Sports Medicine (NASM) Performance Enhancement Specialist, Certified Personal Trainer and Youth Fitness Specialist with the International Youth Conditioning Association (IYCA). He prides himself on being a no-nonsense Fitness Professional who is serious about one thing: achieving your results faster than anyone else.

Tyler's work ethic and dedication to goals and a results-oriented lifestyle is apparent in his own body of work. He earned the honor of a Professional Natural Bodybuilder with the World Natural Bodybuilding Federation (WNBF) in only 3 years of competition and won the 2010 WNBF Mid America Lightweight Championship and finished as the 3rd place Middleweight in the World at the 2010 WNBF World Championships. Tyler prides himself on training more like a world-class athlete than your typical gym going bodybuilder.

In his 5 years in the Farmington Valley area of Connecticut, he has helped well over 400 people change they way they look, feel and move. Having worked in the fitness industry for over 8 years, Tyler continuously saw the same thing occurring at gyms and health clubs: people would repeatedly sign a one or two-year membership with the belief that this was the place they were going to get in shape – when the truth was that many of these soon-to-be frustrated exercisers would end up right back where they started.

Tyler had a vision for a facility that would allow only those seriously committed to creating the lifestyle change that is your personal health and fitness. After the massive success of Farmington Valley Fitness Boot Camp, and its rapid growth in only 2 short months of existence, Tyler English Fitness, Connecticut's Number # 1 Hardcore Gym For Serious Results, was opened.

That vision expanded in August of 2010 when Tyler joined forces with Dr. Joe Klemczewski and became the first Diet Doc Permanent Weight-Loss Program and Clinic in Connecticut. Tyler's fitness industry endeavors didn't stop there, as at the same time he was selected to become the first Athletic Revolution franchisee in the state of Connecticut. Providing youth fitness programming is a natural extension of his commitment to the community.

Tyler earned his Bachelor's Degree in Communications and Marketing from Franklin Pierce College in New Hampshire. While in college, Tyler's love for fitness grew, and he realized his true calling was in the fitness industry. He worked as the Head Strength and Conditioning Consultant at the campus recreation and fitness center, and expanded his work with the pitching staff of the nationally ranked Franklin Pierce

Ravens baseball team.

Upon graduation, Tyler worked in a small handful of gyms and health clubs over a 5-year span before he realized he wanted more. He wanted to create a place where people were always motivated, driven, and would stop at nothing to obtain life-changing results. In 2008, Tyler started out in his mission to change the face of fitness in Farmington Valley.

On January 12th he founded Farmington Valley Fitness Boot Camp. The program has grown to be featured on NBC (Connecticut), FOX and WTNH TV, while helping hundreds of busy men and women from all over Connecticut get into the best shape of their lives.

Tyler has become one of the most respected fitness professionals in the fitness industry – while always displaying a high degree of integrity, responsibility, and ambition. He has proven to be a respected leader within the fitness community, both locally and nationally.

www.TylerEnglishBlog.com
www.TylerEnglishFitness.com
www.FarmingtonValleyFitnessBootCamps.com

Tasha (TK)

while trying to
compose a most wonderful statement
Terry belched (Bighorn sheep imitation)
so I lost my train of thought.
You Rock & Alanta must
love having you!

Marla

Tasha,

It has been at last
having you here. You are a
joy to be around + I have many
happy moments to treasure. I look
forward to hearing your journey + to
reading your goal! You are a winner
Rock on lady!

Jenny.
xx

Tasha,

It was so awesome having you at the fitness adventure and sharing lots of laughs. Keep up your thirst for travel and adventure and good luck with your running goal. Can't wait to keep in touch!

All the best,

Seth Colby

Tasha,
Great to know you, you should know you should be a 'talk show' host! from lady - you are a talk show host! Jacqui

Tasha,
Thank you so much
for your candor. Best wishes
in your progress. Love your humor &
look forward to seeing the butterfly
you become.

Tasha,
It was awesome meeting
you - love your attitude,
hilarious, Good luck with
everything.
KRISTIN

STALIN'S SHADOW

Also by Rosamond Richardson:

SWANBROOKE DOWN
TALKING ABOUT BEREAVEMENT

STALIN'S SHADOW

INSIDE THE FAMILY OF ONE OF THE WORLD'S GREATEST TYRANTS

Rosamond Richardson

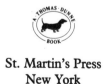

St. Martin's Press
New York

ISBN 0-312-10493-6

First published in Great Britain by Little, Brown and Company Limited.

First U.S. Edition: February 1994
10 9 8 7 6 5 4 3 2 1

ACKNOWLEDGEMENTS

I wish to acknowledge the following writers for quoting short excerpts from their works: Anna Akhmatova, *Selected Poems* (transl. D.M. Thomas), Martin Secker & Warburg Ltd and Penguin, 1988; Milovan Djilas, *Conversations with Stalin*, Penguin, 1962; C.G. Jung, *Psychological reflections* (ed. Jacobi), Routledge & Kegan Paul, 1971 and *Man and his symbols*, Arkana, 1990; Arthur Koestler, *Darkness at Noon*, Penguin, 1947 and *Janus*, Picador, 1978; Alec de Yonge, *Stalin*, Fontana, 1987; Isaac Deutscher, *Stalin*, Penguin, 1966; Brian Masters, *Killing for Company*, Coronet, 1986; Eugeny Yevtushenko, *Autobiography*, Flegon Press, 1966; Svetlana Alliluyeva, *20 letters to a Friend*, Hutchinson, 1967.

Permission from Michael Joseph to quote at length from *The Alliluyev Memoirs*, ed. David Tutaev, 1968, is gratefully acknowledged by the author. So is the expert editing of Sheila McIlwraith on the completed manuscript. It is difficult to thank Alan Samson sufficiently for his unfailing support, enthusiasm and constructive help during the writing of the book.

Thanks, too, to Alan Bookbinder who worked as my interpreter for the interviews with the Alliluyev family in Moscow, and who steered me skilfully around the capital. His intelligent support was much appreciated.

My thanks above all to Svetlana Alliluyeva, Stalin's daughter, without whose help this book neither would nor could have been written, for the many hours spent in conversation with her, for the Moscow contacts, for her collection of family photographs, and for the warmth and friendship shared during the preparation of this book. I am indebted to her for the form that it has taken, and for numerous intimate insights into the life of her family.

Note
The adaptation of Stalin's first name *Iosif* to Joseph has been used in this book because of its world-wide familiarity. All the other Russian names have simply been transliterated.

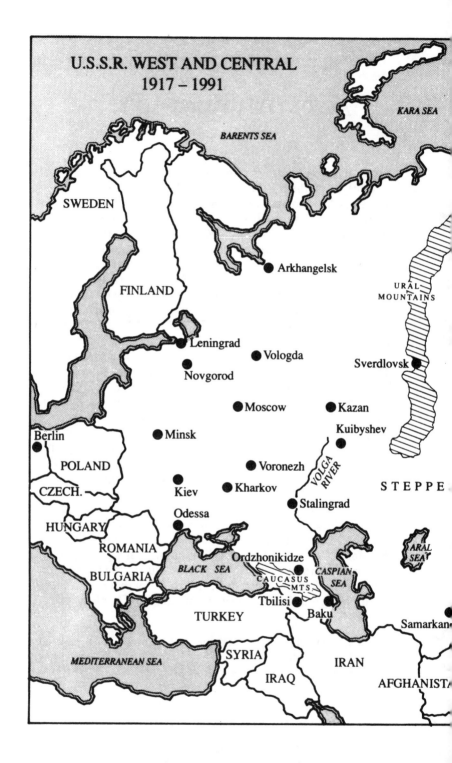

U.S.S.R. WEST AND CENTRAL
1917 – 1991

KARA SEA

BARENTS SEA

SWEDEN

FINLAND

● Arkhangelsk

URAL
MOUNTAINS

● Leningrad

● Vologda

Sverdlovsk ●

● Novgorod

● Moscow

● Kazan

Berlin
●

● Minsk

Kuibyshev
●

POLAND

● Voronezh

VOLGA RIVER

S T E P P E

CZECH.

● Kiev

● Kharkov

● Stalingrad

HUNGARY

● Odessa

ARAL SEA

ROMANIA

Ordzhonikidze
●

CASPIAN SEA

BULGARIA

BLACK   SEA

C A U C A S U S
M T S

● Tbilisi

● Baku

● Samarkand

TURKEY

SYRIA

IRAN

MEDITERRANEAN SEA

IRAQ

AFGHANISTAN

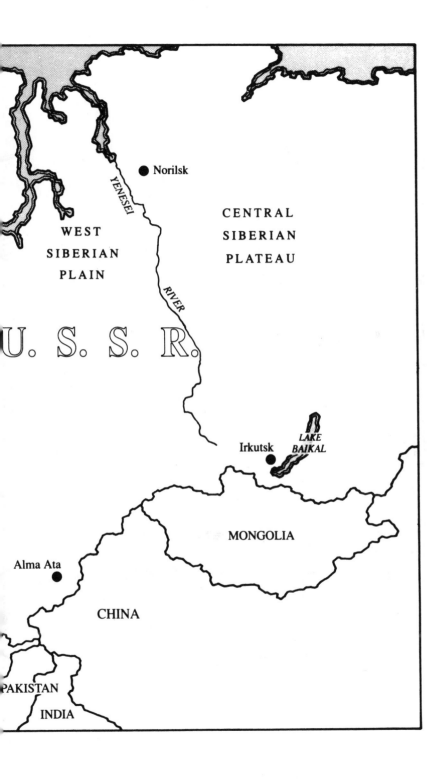

THE DJUGASHVILI (STALIN) FAMILY TREE

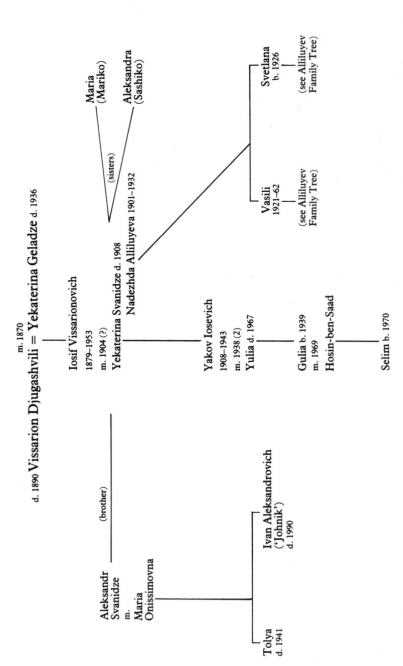

THE ALLILUYEV FAMILY TREE

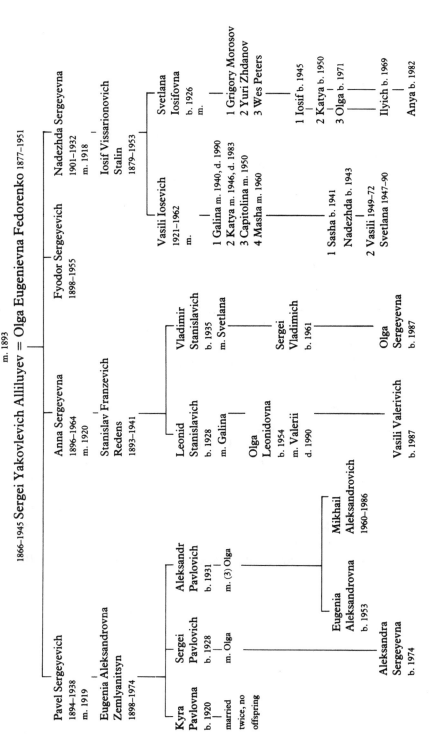